EAR Acupuncture

CLINICAL TREATMENT

耳穴临床疗法

Sumiko Knudsen

Ph.D
Practitioner, DK

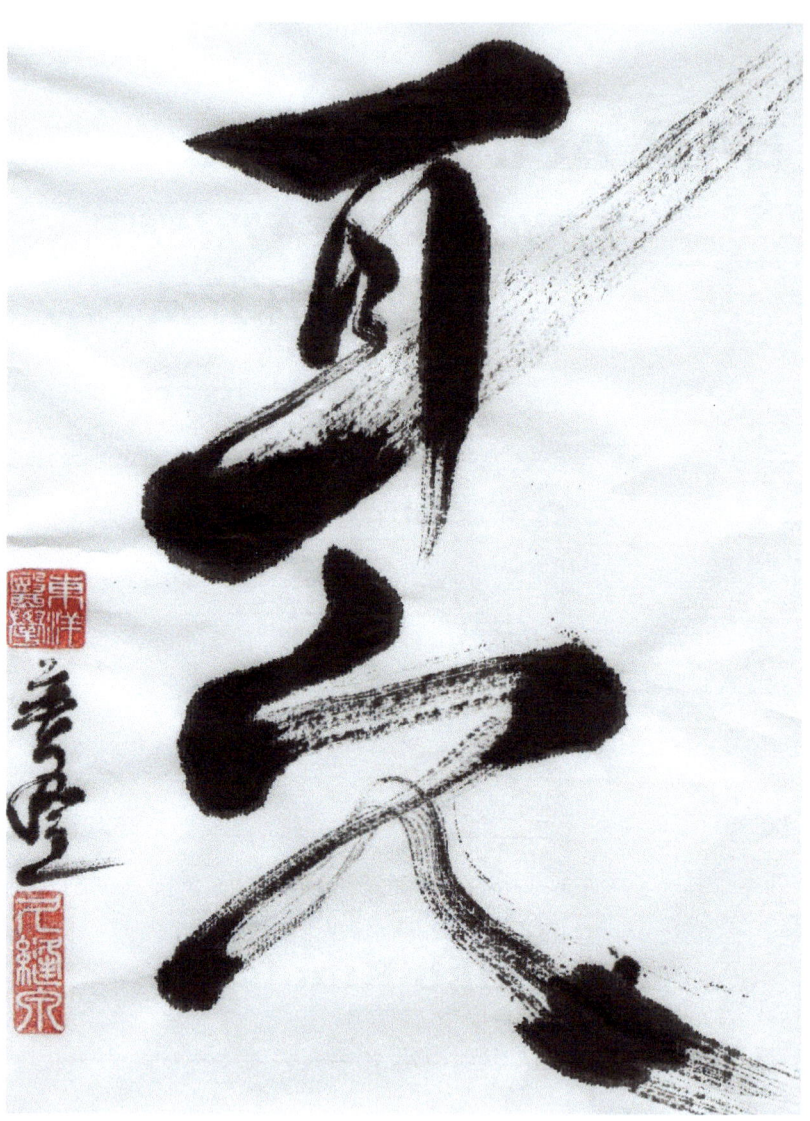

Forlag: BoD – Books on Demand, København, Danmark
Tryk: BoD – Books on Demand, Norderstedt, Tyskland

ISBN: 9788743016298

CONTENTS

INTRODUCTION

Ear (Auricular) acupuncture therapy has been widely used and practiced in many countries in the world. It has quickly become to recognize by patients, and one of the benefits is, it is provided easily application while patients are seated or lay down. Therefore, it is good to combine body acupuncture and ear acupuncture.

Ear (Auricular) acupuncture points are different from acupuncture meridians and points. The ear is a micro system, which reflects the entire body, represented on the ear.

Ear (Auricular) acupuncture points are used on independent and specific organs in zones where the stimulation is applied for prevention and treatment of diseases.

Ear points are tightly connected with human body organs and systems with body channels according to the traditional Chinese Medicine.

Ear (Auricular) acupuncture is effective for many diseases and has recorded the effectiveness in many countries.

Ear points in use recognized by WHO.

Sumiko Knudsen 克努森澄子

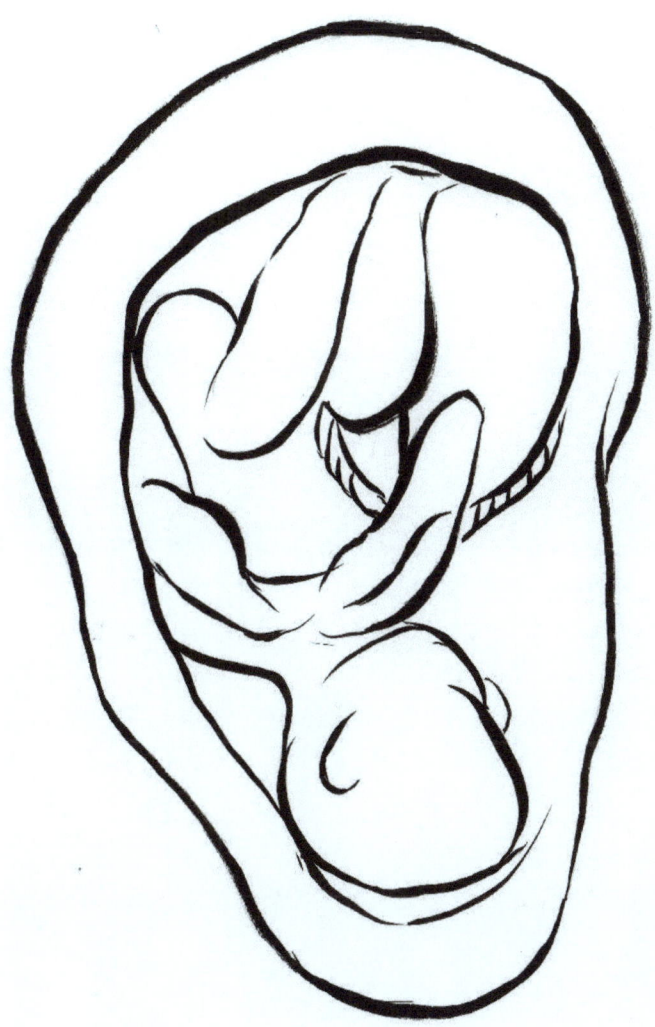

Fetus map on the external ear

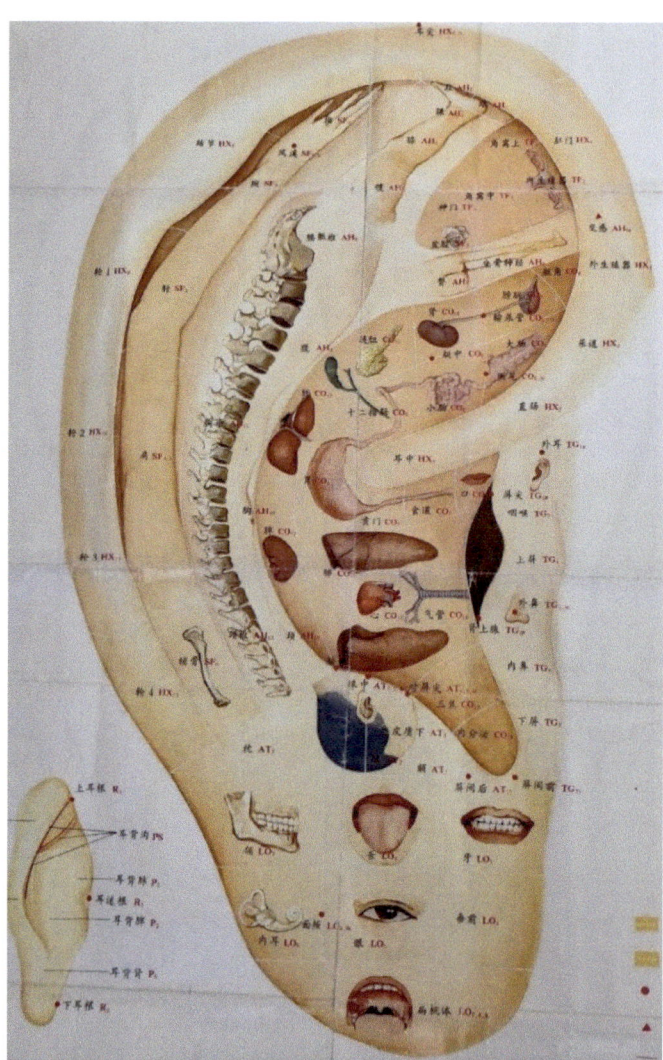

Standard Auricular points

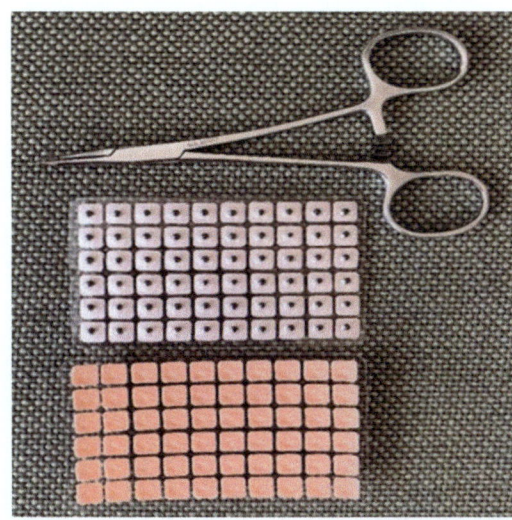

Ear vaccaria seeds

Ear acupoint diagnosis apparatus

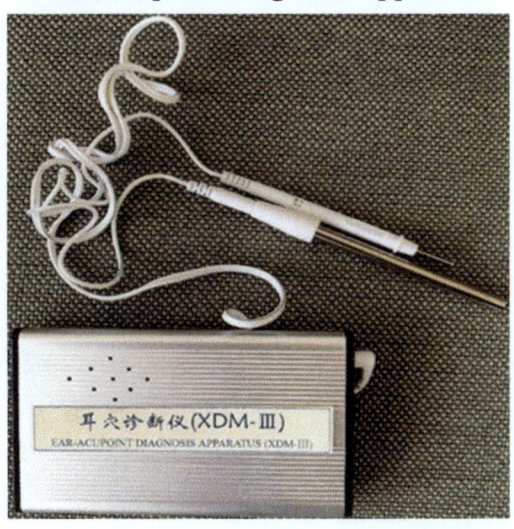

I. Anatomical Structure of the Auricular Surface

To facilitate location of Ear Points, Anatomical Structures of the Auricular surface relating to Ear Acupuncture are as follows.

1. Helix 耳
2. Helix Tubercle 耳轮结节
3. Helix Cauda 耳轮尾
4. Helix Crus 耳轮脚
5. Antihelix 对耳轮
6. The principal part of Antihelix 对耳轮体
7. Superior Antihelix Crus 对耳轮上脚
8. Inferior Antihelix Crus 对耳轮下脚
9. Triangular Fossa 三角窝
10. Scapha 耳舟
11. Tragus 耳屏
12. Supratragic Notch 屏上切迹
13. Antitragus 对耳屏
14. Intertragic Notch 屏间切迹
15. Helix Notch 轮屏切迹
16. Ear Lobe 耳垂
17. Concha 甲腔
18. Cymba Concha 耳甲艇
19. Cavity Concha 耳甲腔

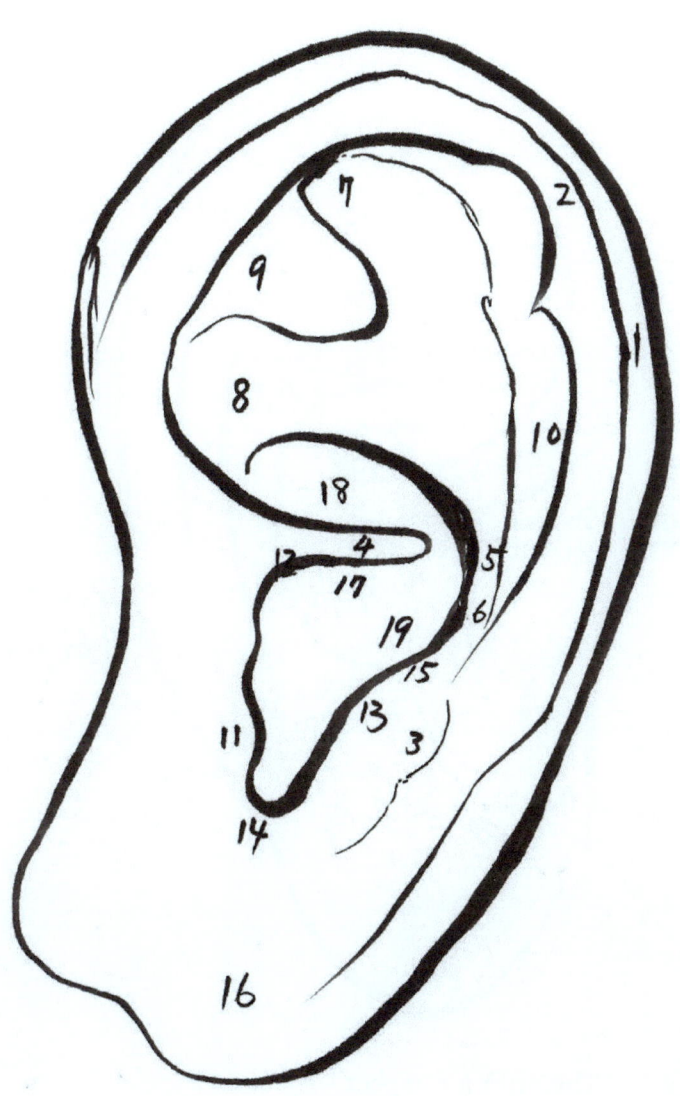

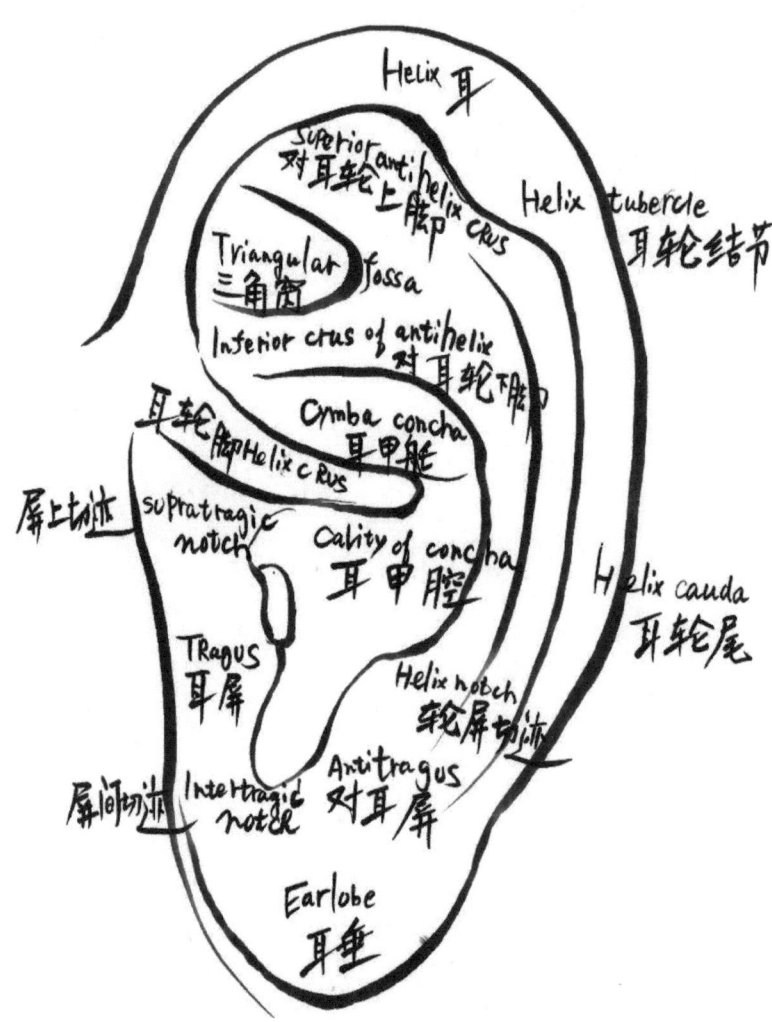

The anterior aspect

II. Auricular Points

Auricular points are specific stimulating points on the ear. When the disorder occurs in the parts of the body, then it may appear various reactions at the corresponding areas of the ear. Thus, in order to make a diagnosis, it can be taken to stimulate the sensitive sites, and to prevent diseases.

1.The Corresponding Regional Anatomy of the Acupuncture Points

1.1. Distribution of Ear Points

The distribution of ear points on the ear follows a certain scheme.

The ear is compared to an inverted fetus with the head down towards the top. Ear points corresponding to head and face are near Earlobe. The points corresponding to the upper limbs are at the Scapha. Lower limbs are around the superior and inferior crus of Antihelix. Internal organs are Cymba Concha and Cavity of Concha.

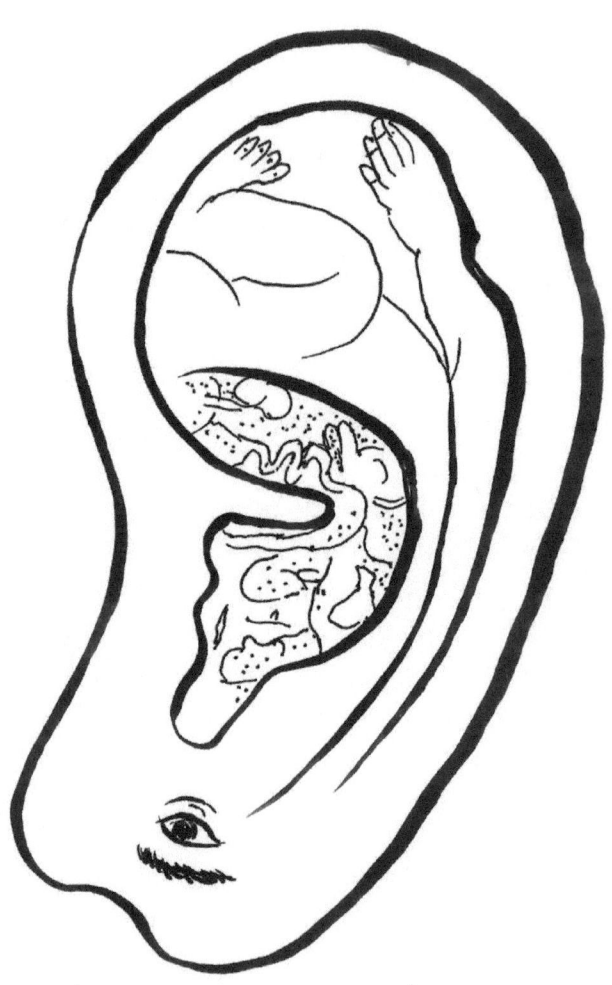

1.1.   Ear Points for the distribution pattern

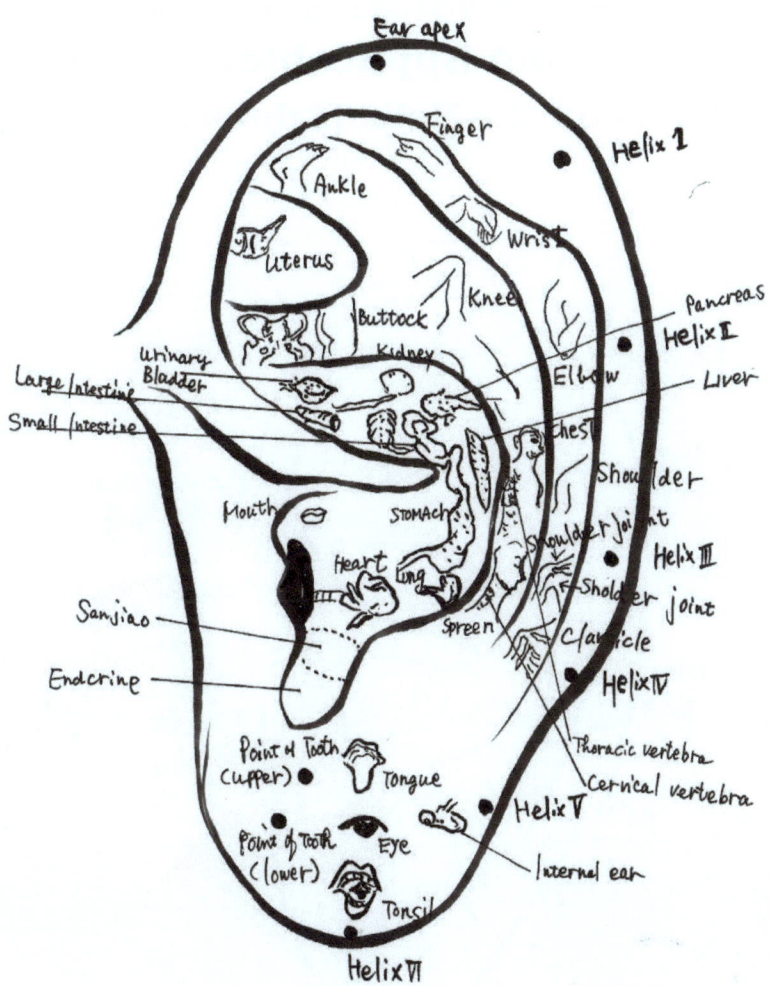

1.2.   Ear Points for the corresponding regional anatomy

III. Auricular points Location, Function and Applicable Disease
1. Points on the Helix (Erlunxuewei 耳轮穴位)

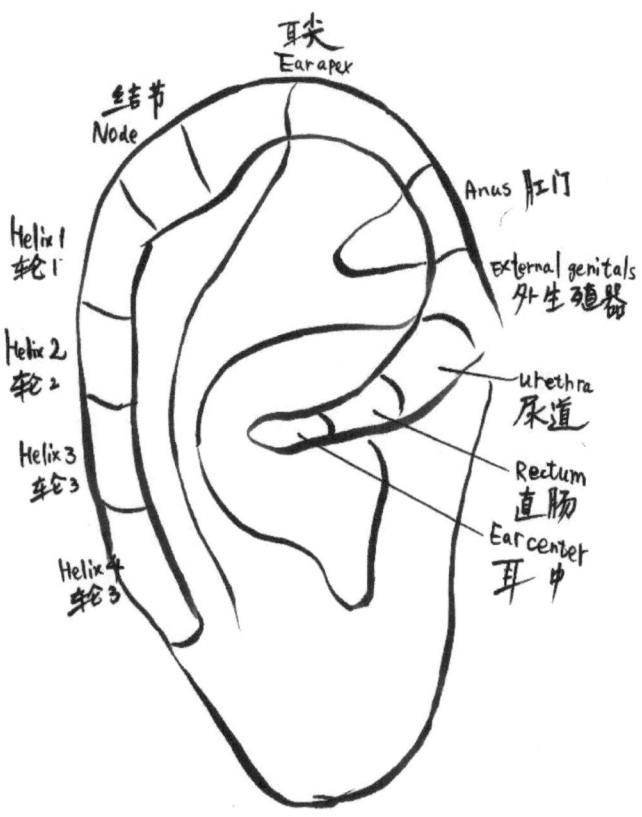

1. Ear Center (Erzhong 耳中)

Location: On the Helix.
Function: Relax muscular spasm.
Control Qi, Blood circulation and dispel wind and relieve pain.
Treatment:Hiccup, Vomiting, Blood deficiency/stasis/heat, hemorrhage, metrorrhagia.

2. Rectum (Zhichang 直肠)

Location: On the Helix.
Function: Laxation and alleviate diarrhea.
Treatment:Constipation, Diarrhea, prolapse anus, Hemorrhoid.

3. Urethra (Niaodao 尿道)

Location: On the Helix.
Function: Heat away and dampness. Relieve the muscular spasm and pain.
Treatment:Bed-wetting, frequent urination, painful urination, pruritis of the genitals.

4. External genitals (Waishengzhiqi 外生殖器)

Location: On the Helix.
Function: Clear heat and dampness in Liver and Gallbladder. Clear blood heat, dispel wind, relieve itching for sexual function.
Treatment: Various genitals diseases.
Testitis, vaginitis, itching vulvae.

5. Anus (Gangmen 肛门)

Location: On the Helix.
Function: Clear heat and relieve swelling and pain. Promote laxation and blood flow.
Treatment: Prolapse anus, hemorrhoid.

6. Ear apex (Erjian 耳尖)

Location: On the top of the Helix.
Function: Clear heat and remove toxic substance. Calm liver, cool blood, relieve itching and swelling pain.
Treatment: Hypertension, fever, Eye disease, eczema, urticaria.

7. Node (Jiejie 结节)

Location: On the tubercle of the Helix.
Function: Clear heat and toxic in Liver.

Relieve the depressed Liver and regulate the circulation of Qi.

Treatment: Hepatitis, Headache, dizziness.

Pain around the waist and armpit of the body region.

8. Helix 1 (Lunyi1 轮 1)
9. Helix 2 (Lunyi2 轮 2)
10.Helix 3 (Lunyi3 轮 3)
11.Helix 4 (Lunyi4 轮 4)

Location: On the Helix.

Function: Clear heat and remove toxic substances.

Treatment: Cold, respiratory tract infection, tonsillitis. Clear heat and various inflammation of syndrome.

2. Points on the Scapha (Erzhou 耳舟)

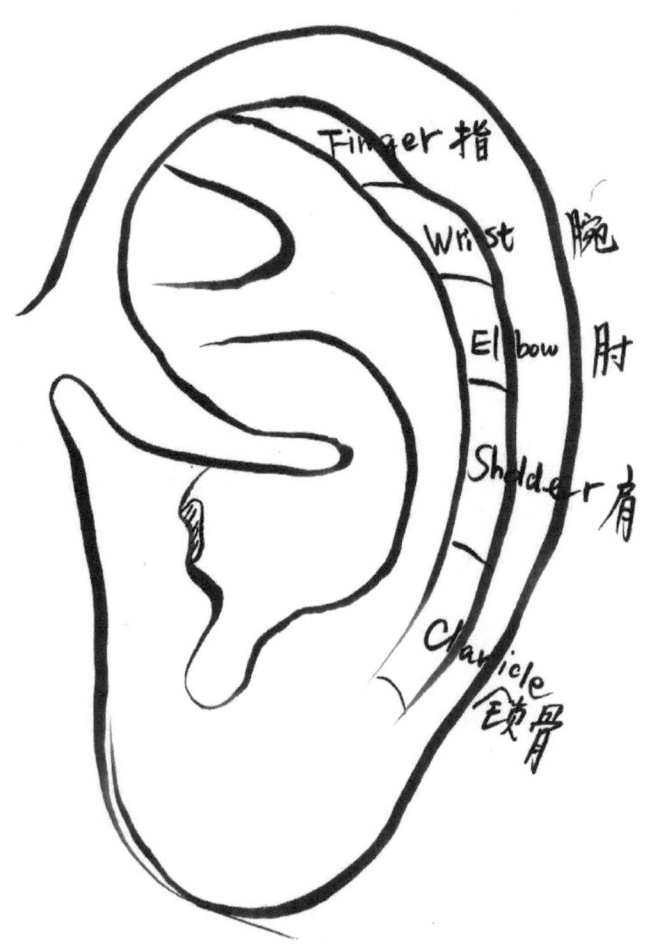

1. Finger (Zhi 指)

Location: On the uppermost part of the Scaphoid fossa.

Function: Promote the blood circulation, dispel the wind, relieve pain and inflammation.

Treatment: Pain, numbness, sprain of the finger joint.

2. Wrist (Wan 腕)

Location: Inferior to the finger point.

Function: Promote the blood circulation, dispel the wind, relieve pain.

Treatment: Wrist pain sprain the wrist joint.

3. Wind stream (Fengxi 风溪)

Location: Between the finger point and wrist.

Function: Promote the blood flow, dispel the wind and itching, relieve cough and asthma.

Treatment: Asthma, allergic rhinitis and colitis, acne, urticaria, eczema.

3. Elbow (Zhou 肘)

Location: Inferior to the wrist point.

Function: Promote the blood flow. Dispel the wind. Relieve the pain.

Treatment: Elbow pain, tennis elbow, sprain elbow joint and rheumatic arthritis.

4. Shoulder (Jian 肩)

Location: Inferior to the elbow point.

Function: Promote the blood flow. Dispel the wind. Relieve the pain.

Treatment: Shoulder pain, sprain of shoulder joint, upper limbs dysfunction, pain by cervical spondylosis.

5. Clavicle (Suogu 锁骨)

Location: Inferior to the shoulder point.

Function: Dispel the wind, clear the dampness. Relieve the pain.

Treatment: Shoulder pain, back pain, neck pain, rheumatic pain, stiff neck.

3. Points on the Antihelix
(Duierlunxuewei 对耳轮穴位)

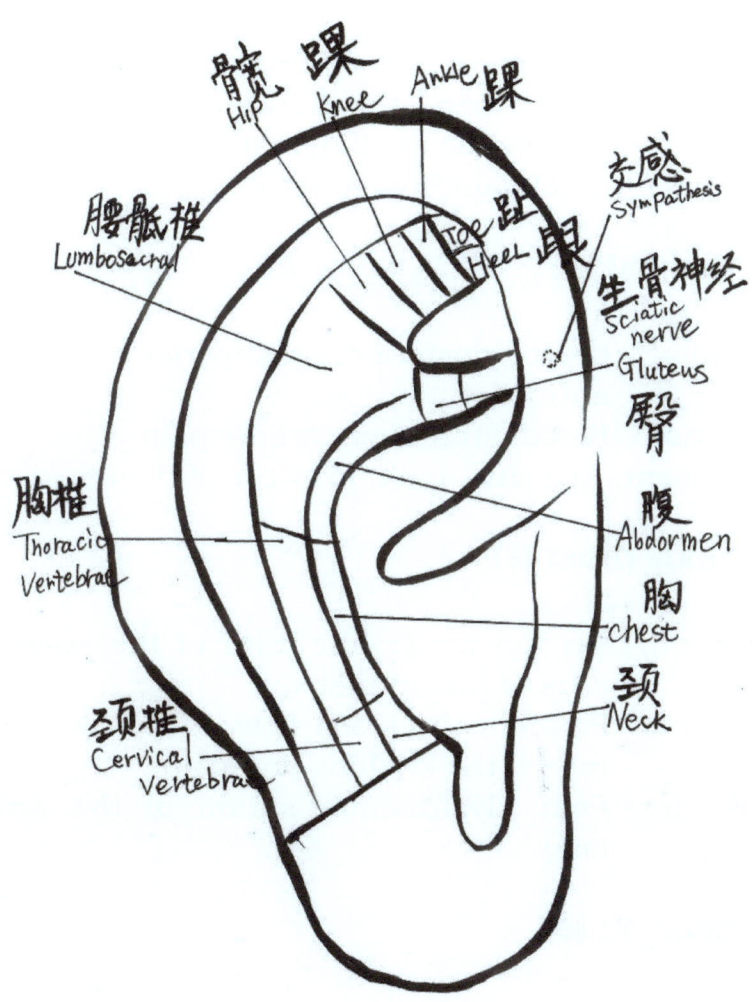

1. Heel (Gen 跟)

Location: On the anterior and superior crus of the antihelix.
Function: Promote the blood flow, dispel the wind. Strengthen the muscles and bones. Relieve the swelling and pain.
Treatment: Heel pain, injury swelling etc.

2. Toe (Zhi 趾)

Location: On the posterior and superior crus of the antihelix.
Function: Blood circulation, relieve pain.
Treatment: Arthritis, pain, pruritus of the toe joints.

3. Ankle (Huai 踝)

Location: On the upper one-third of the superior crus of the antihelix.
Function: Promote the blood flow, dispel the wind relieve the swelling and pain.
Treatment: Pain, dysfunction sprain of the ankle joint.

4. Knee (Xi 膝)

Location: On the middle one-third of the superior crus.
Function: Dispel the wind, clear the dampness and relieve pain.
Treatment: Swelling and pain of knee joint , rheumatic arthritis, sprain of the knee joint.

5. Hip (Kuan 髋)

Location: On the lower one-third of the superior crus of the antihelix.
Function: Promote the blood flow, dispel the wind relieve pain.
Treatment: Sciatic nerve, lumbosacral pain, arthritis.

6. Sciatic nerv (Zuogushenjing 坐骨神经)

Location: On the anterior two-thirds of the inferior crus.
Function: Strengthen the muscles and bones, relieve pain.
Treatment: Sciatica, paralysis of the lower limbs.

7. Sympathesis (Jiaogan 交感)

Location: Crus of the antihelix and the internal
            edge of the Helix.
Function: Relax of the spasm of the muscle. Treat
            the visceral pain.
Treatment: Insomnia, hyperhidrosis neurosis of
            visceral organs, asthma, gastric ulcer,
            visceral colic.

8. Gluteus (Tun 臀)

Location: On the posterior one-third of the inferior
            crus.
Function: Promote the blood flow, dispel the wind,
            relieve pain.
Treatment: Sciatica, buttocks and sacral pain.

9. Abdomen (Fu 腹)

Location: On the anterior and superior two-fifths of
            the antihelix.
Function: Muscular spasm relieve pain.
Treatment: Abdominal pain and distension, diarrhea,
            constipation, lumbar sprain,
            gallstone, dysmenorrhea, irregular
            menstruation.

10. Lumbosacral vertebrae (Yaodizhui 腰骶椎)

Location: On the posterior of the abdomen.

Function: Promote the blood flow, relieve pain. Strengthen the bone. Reinforce bone.

Treatment: Lumbosacral pain, dysfunction of lower limbs, lumber muscle strain, numbness of lower limbs, rheumatoid arthritis. Urinary incontinence, sciatica.

11. Chest (Xiong 胸)

Location: On middle and anterior two-fifths of the antihelix.

Function: Regulate Qi and alleviate depression.

Treatment: Heart disease, Zoster, costal chondritis, intercostal neuralgia.

12. Thoracic vertebrae (Xiongzhui 胸椎)

Location: Posterior to the chest point.

Function: Promote the blood flow, dispel the wind, relieve pain.

Treatment: Chest and back pain, back muscles strain, intercostal neuralgia.

13.Neck (Jing 颈)

Location: On the anterior and inferior one-fifth of the antihelix.
Function: Regulate thyroid function.
Treatment:Stiff neck, cervical sprain, thyroid swelling, hyperthyroidism.

14.Cervical vertebrae (Jingzhui 颈椎)

Location: Posterior to the neck point.
Function: Promote the blood flow, dispel window, strengthen the muscles and bones, relieve the pain.

Treatment:Stiff neck, rheumatoid arthritis, paralysis of the upper limbs, itching, thyroid enlargement.

4. Points on the Triangular Fossa (sanjiaowoxuewei 三角窝穴位)

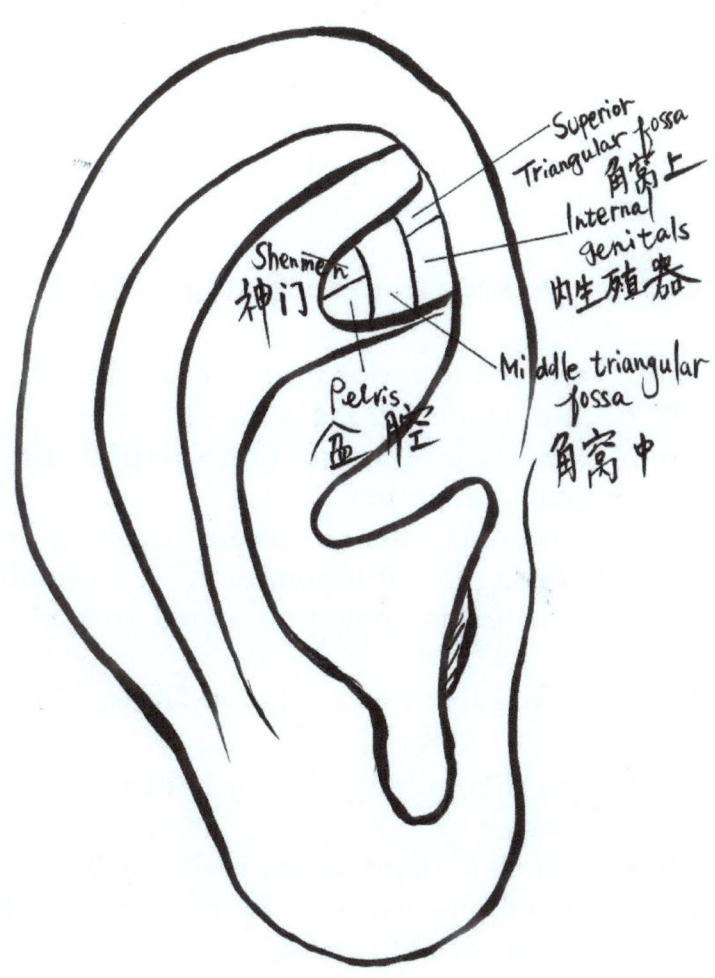

1. Superior triangular fossa (Jiaowoshang 角窝上)

Location: On the anterior and superior one-third of triangular fossa.
Function: Decrease the blood pressure, regulate and nourish the Liver and Kidney, nourish the blood.
Treatment:Hypertension, headache, vertigo.

2. Internal genitals (Neishengzhiqi 内生殖器)

Location: On the anterior and inferior one-third of the triangular fossa.
Function: Regulate menstruation, nourish Kidney, pelvic infection.
Treatment:Irregular menstruation, dysmenorrhea, pelvic inflammation, impotence prostatitis, male and female infertility.

3. Middle triangular fossa (Jiaowozhong 角窝中)

Location: On the middle one-third of the triangular fossa.
Function: Alleviate depression, regulate Qi.
Treatment:Bronchial asthma, fullness of the chest, shortness of breath.

4. Shenmen (神门)

Location: On the posterior and superior one-third of the triangular fossa.
Function: Relieve muscular spasm, pain, and inflammation. Calm Liver.
Treatment:(1) Hypertension.
         (2) urticaria, eczema, cough.
         (3) headache, inflammation.

5. Pelvis (Penqiang 盆腔)

Location: On the posterior and inferior one-third of the triangular fossa.
Function: Clear heat and dampness. Relieve pain.
Treatment:Pelvic inflammation, prostatitis, irregular menstruation, lower limb pain, abdominal pain.

5. Points on the Tragus (Erpingxuewei 耳屏穴位)

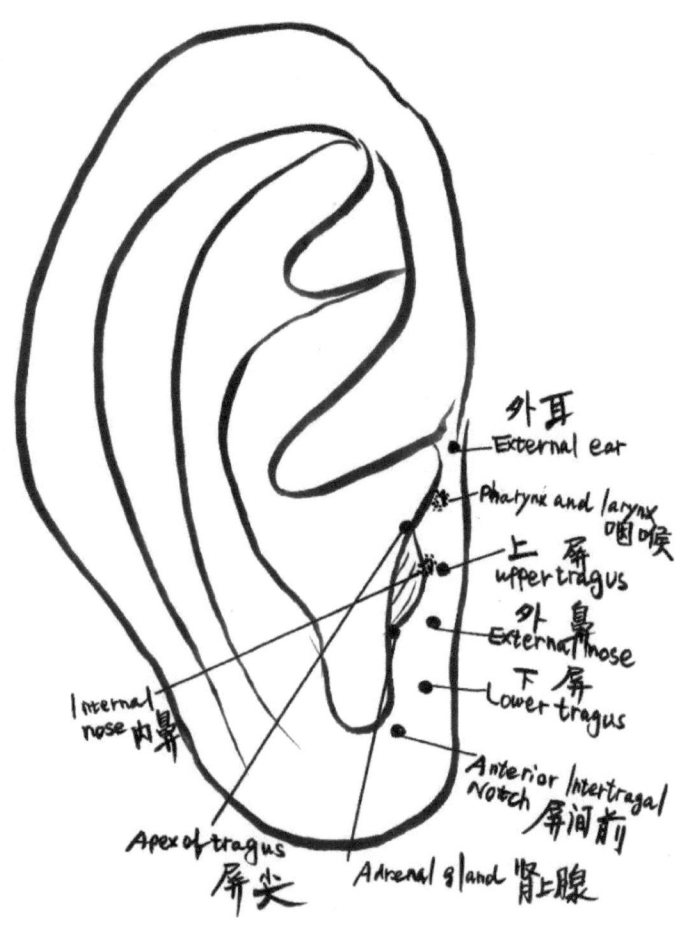

外耳
External ear

Pharynx and larynx 咽喉

上 屏
upper tragus

外 鼻
External nose

下 屏
Lower tragus

Internal nose 内鼻

Anterior Intertragal Notch 屏间前

Apex of tragus 屏尖

Adrenal gland 肾上腺

1. External ear (Waier 外耳)

Location: On the upper edge of the tragus.
Function: Promote blood circulation, clear the blood stasis, calm down and relieve pain.
Treatment: Dizziness, migraine, deafness and tinnitus, cervical pain.

2. Apex of the tragus (Pingjian 屏尖)

Location: On the posterior edge of the tragus.
Function: Anti-inflammation, reduce fever, tranquil pain.
Treatment: Toothache, Fever, inflammation, pain.

3. External nose (Waibi 外鼻)

Location: The center of the external edge of the tragus.
Function: Clear heat, promote the blood flow, relieve pain.
Treatment: Rhinitis, nasal obstruction.

4. Adrenal gland (Shenshangxian 肾上腺)

Location: On the apex of the inferior tragus.

Function: Anti-infection relieves cough and asthma, anti-rheumatism, coordinate the function of adrenal gland.
Treatment:(1) Rheumatic arthritis.
(2) Allergic disease, asthma, cough, inflammations.
(3) Hemorrhagic disease, hypotension.

5. Pharynx and larynx (Yanhou 咽喉)

Location: On the superior of the internal side of the tragus.
Function: Expel toxin, relieve inflammation and swelling, resolve sputum and clear the throat.
Treatment: Pharyngitis, tonsillitis, hoarseness, bronchitis, bronchial asthma.

6. Internal nose (Neibi 内鼻)

Location: On the inferior half of the internal of the tragus.
Function: Dispel wind, stop bleeding.
Treatment:Cold, nasal obstruction, rhinitis, epistaxis.

7. Anterior intertragal notch (Pingjianqian 屏间前)

Location: On the lowest part of the tragus, on the inferior edge of the tragus.
Function: Clear heat, promote blood circulation, clear the heat in brain for brightening eyes.
Treatment: Dizziness, headache, glaucoma, myopia, retinitis.

6.Points on the Antitragus
(Duierpingxuewei 对耳屏穴位)

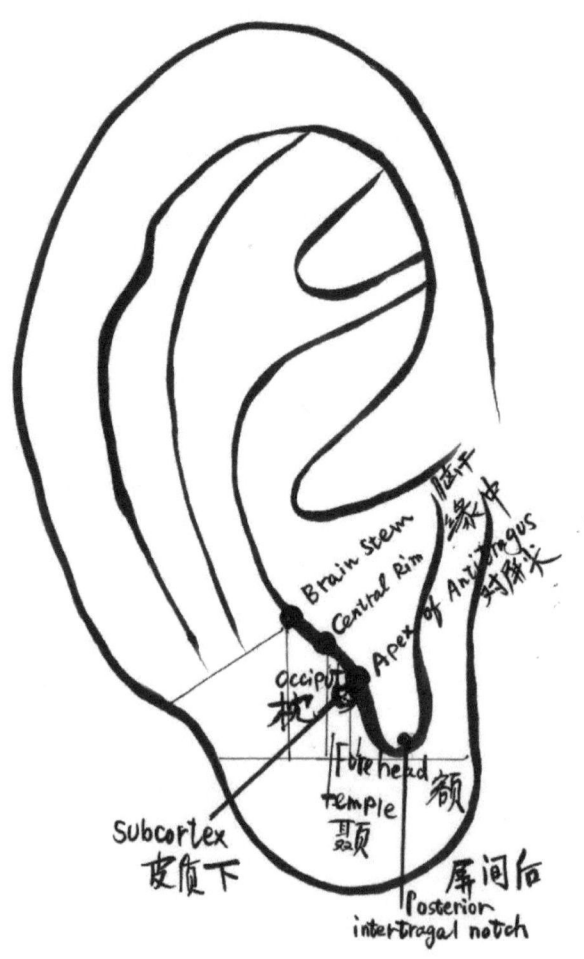

1. Forehead (E 额)

Location: On the anterior part of the antitragus.
Function: Strengthen the function of brain and brighten eyes.
Treatment: Dizziness, insomnia, myopia, sinusitis, rhinitis.

2. Posterior intertragal notch (Pingjianhou 屏间后)

Location: Posterior to the notch between tragus and antitragus, on the inferior edge of the antitragus.
Function: Relieve the heat and toxin, cool the blood, brighten the eyes.
Treatment: Glaucoma, stye, eye disease.

3. Temple (Nie 颞)

Location: On the middle of the external side of the antitragus.
Function: Regulate Qi, relieve Liver and Gallbladder, brighten eye, relieve tinnitus.
Treatment: Dizziness, migraine, tinnitus.

4. Occiput (Zhen 枕)

Location: On the posterior of the external side of the antitragus.

Function: Clear heat, dispel itching, relieve cough and asthma, brighten eyes.

Treatment:(1) Dizziness, headache, seasickness.
(2) Meningitis, brain trauma,
(3) Insomnia.
(4) Asthma.

5. Subcortex (Pizhixia 皮质下)

Location: On the medial side of the antitragus.

Function: dispel pain, relieve hiccup and vomiting, nourish the brain and calm the mind.

Treatment:(1) Gastritis, nausea, vomiting, abdominal distension, constipation, hiccup.
(2) Insomnia, dreaminess.

6. Apex of the antitragus (Duipingjian 对屏尖)

Location: On the apex of antitragus.

Function: Relieve cough and asthma, dispel itching.

Treatment:Cough, asthma, short breath, pruritus.

7. Central rim (Yuanzhong 缘中)

Location: On the antitragus, junction among the antitragus.

Function: Relieve muscular spasm, nourish the brain.

Treatment: Vertigo, cerebral concussion.

8. Brain stem (Naogan 脑干)

Location: On the antitragus, between antitragus and antihelix.

Function: Relieve muscular spasm, replenish the brain.

Treatment: Epilepsy, schizophrenia, neurosis, vertigo, headache.

7.Points on the Concha (Erjiaxuewei 耳甲穴位)

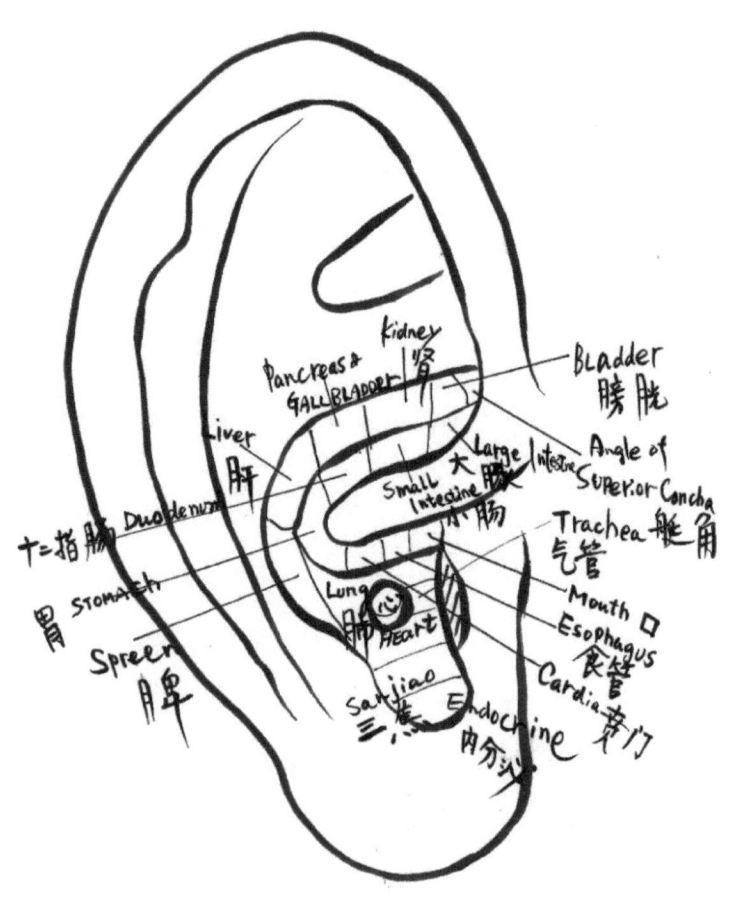

1. Mouth (Kou 口)

Location: On the anterior one-third of the concha, under the inferior crus of the antihelix.
Function: Relieve muscular spasm, cough, asthma and pain. Regulate gastrointestinal function.
Treatment: Bronchial asthma, cough, insomnia, oral ulcer, facial paralysis.

2. Esophagus (Shidao 食道)

Location: On the middle one-third of the concha.
Function: Treat dysphagia, promote appetite, regulate esophagus.
Treatment: Chest distress, short breath, difficult to fall asleep.

3. Cardia (Penmen 喷门)

Location: On the anterior one-third of the concha.
Function: Relieve spasm, regulate stomach, promote appetite.
Treatment: Nausea, cardio spasm, vomiting, chest discomfort.

4. Stomach (Wei 胃)

Location: On the terminus of the superior crus of the helix.

Function: Regulate the flow of Qi, invigorate Spleen, relieve vomiting and pain.

Treatment (1) Gastric ulcer gastrointestinal dysfunction.

5. Duoderum (Shierzhichang 十二指肠)

Location: On the posterior one-third of the inferior crus of the helix.

Function: Relieve spasm and pain, regulate gastrointestinal function.

Treatment: Abdominal distension, diarrhea, cholecystitis.

6. Small intestine (Xiaochang 小肠)

Location: On the middle one-third of the superior crus of the helix.

Function: Clear dampness and heat, relieve diarrhea, promote circulation of Qi and remove obstruction. Eliminate heat.

Treatment: Diarrhea, abdominal distension, intestinal tuberculosis.

7. Large intestine (Dachang 大肠)

Location: On the anterior one-third of the inferior crus.
Function: Remove heat, relieve cough, diarrhea.
Treatment: Diarrhea, intestinal dysfunction. Cough asthma, cold pneumonia respiratory tract disease, acne.

8. Appendix (Lanwei 阑尾)

Location: Between the point of Large intestine and Small intestine.
Function: Clear heat, promote blood circulation.
Treatment: Diarrhea. Appendicitis.

9. Angle of superior concha (Tingjiao 艇角)

Location: On the anterior of the concha, inferior to the inferior crus.
Function: Nourish Kidney, eliminate dampness, promote blood circulation, eliminate stagnation and remove abdominal mass.
Treatment: Bronchial asthma, Epistaxis.

10. Bladder (Pangguang 膀胱)

Location: On the middle of the concha inferior to the inferior crus of the helix.

Function: Relieve heat and dampness, regulate Qi circulation, relieve pain.

Treatment: Backache, spinal column pain, sciatica.

11. Kidney (Shen 肾)

Location: On the posterior of the concha inferior to the inferior crus of the helix.

Function: Nourish Yin and strengthen Yang of Kidney, strengthen the back, improve eyesight.

Treatment: Heel and leg pain, dizziness, insomnia, brain and spinal marrow, rheumatoid arthritis.

12. Ureter (Shuniaoguan 输尿管)

Location: Between Kidney and Bladder.

Function: Clear heat and dampness in lower Jiao, relax spasm.

Treatment: Urinary infections.

13. Pancreas and gallbladder (Yidan 胰胆)

Location: On the posterior and superior of the superior concha.
Function: Disperse the depressed Qi of Liver and Gallbladder. Relieve pain.
Treatment: (1) Cholecystitis, fullness of hypochondriac region.
(2) Diabetes mellitus, insomnia, tinnitus, migræne.

14. Liver (Gan 肝)

Location: On the posterior and inferior part.
Function: Smooth Liver, Qi and blood circulation, remove blood stasis.
Treatment: (1) Hepatitis.
(2) Dysfunctional menstruation, dysmenorrhea, dizziness, gynecologic diseases.
(3) Muscle spasm, limb numbness convulsion of hand and foot

15. Center of superior concha (Tingzhong 艇中)

Location: Between the Small Intestine and Kidney.

Function: Regulate of Qi circulation, relieve pain.
Treatment: Abdominal pain and distension.

16. Spleen (Pi 脾)

Location: On the posterior and superior of the inferior concha.
Function: Clear dampness and heat, raise Qi, function of digestion and transportation.
Treatment:Edema, stagnation of phlegm and dampness, hemorrhagic syndrome, metrorrhagia, metrostaxis, uterine bleeding.

17. Heart (Xin 心)

Location: On the central and the inferior concha.
Function: Eliminate heart-fire, clear blood stasis
Treatment:(1) Heart disease, neurosis, insomnia, dreaminess, night sweating.
(2) hoarseness, pharyngitis.
(3) Skin diseases.

18. Trachea (Qiguan 气管)

Location: Locates side of heart.
Function: Relieve cough and sputum, asthma and sore throat. Expel wind.

Treatment: Bronchial asthma, cold, cough, pharyngitis.

19. Lung (Fei 肺)

Location: Around the heart and trachea.
Function: Promote Qi circulation. Eliminate wind and itching. Relieve cough, asthma.
Treatment: Respiratory diseases, bronchitis, bronchial asthma, palpitation, short breath, oppressed feeling in chest, cough.

20. Sanjiao (三焦)

Location: Posterior and inferior to the canal, between Lung and Endocrine point.
Function: Coordinate the function of Zang Fu organs, Qi circulation, regulate spleen, nourish heart and lung, invigorate kidney.
Treatment: (1) Coronary heart disease, hypochondriac pain short breath.
(2) Edema
(3) Tinnitus, deafness
(4) Pain of the lateral side of the upper limbs.

21. Endocrine (Neifenmi 内分泌)

Location: Inside the notch between the tragus and antitragus.

Function: Anti-infection, promote the blood flow, relieve dampness.

Treatment: Dysmenorrhea, menopausal syndrome, obesity, irregular menstruation, hyperthyroidism.

8.Points on the Earlobe (Erchuixuewei 耳垂穴位)

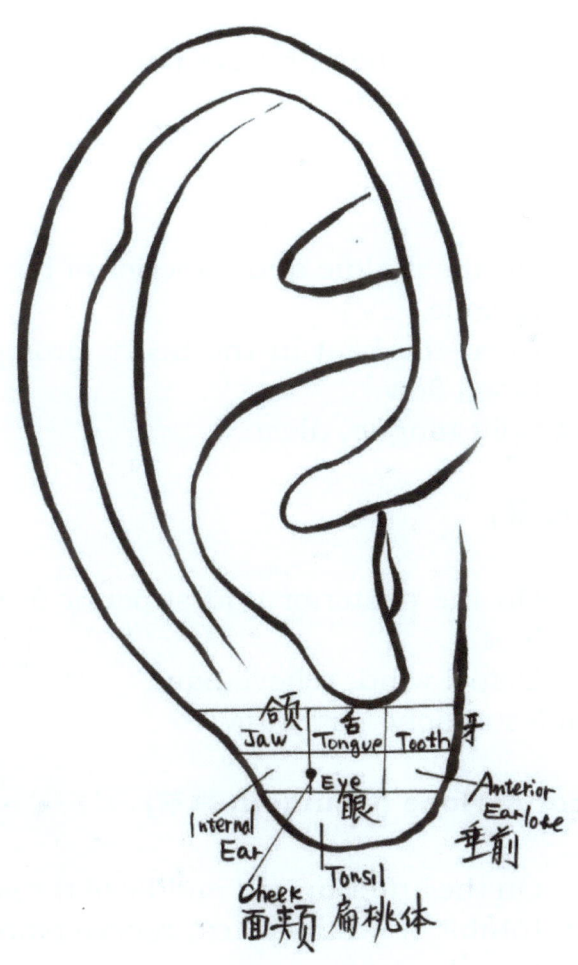

1. Teeth (Ya 牙)

Location: On the anterior and superior of the earlobe.
Function: Clear the heat, relieve pain.
Treatment: Hypotension.

2. Tongue (She 舌)

Location: On the middle and superior of the earlobe.
Function: Clear the heat in the heart, promote the blood flow.
Treatment: Split tongue, ulcer.

3. Jaw (He 颌)

Location: On the posterior and superior of the ear lobe.
Function: Dispel wind, relieve pain.
Treatment: Toothache, arthritis.

4. Anterior earlobe (Chuiqian 垂前)

Location: On the anterior and middle of the earlobe.
Function: Inhibit of brain cortex, relieve pain.

Treatment: Dizziness, insomnia, dreaminess, palpitation.

5. Eye (Yan 眼)

Location: On the center of the earlobe.
Function: Clear heat. Smooth Qi circulation in liver and bright eyes.
Treatment: Conjunctivitis, glaucoma, cataract, myopia, optic atrophy.

6. Internal ear (Neier 内耳)

Location: On the posterior and middle portion of the earlobe.
Function: Dispel wind and heat, improve the function of hearing.
Treatment: Deafness, tinnitus.

7. Cheek (Mianjia 面颊)

Location: Between the eye and internal ear.
Function: Dispel the wind, the spasm. Relieve swelling.
Treatment: Bell's palsy, acne, facial wrinkles.

8. Tonsil (Biantaoti 扁桃体)

Location: On the inferior portion of the earlobe.
Function: Clear heat and toxin, anti-inflammation,
           relieve swelling.
Treatment:Tonsillitis, pharyngitis.

9. Points on the Posterior Surface of the Auricle (Erbeixuewei 耳背穴位)

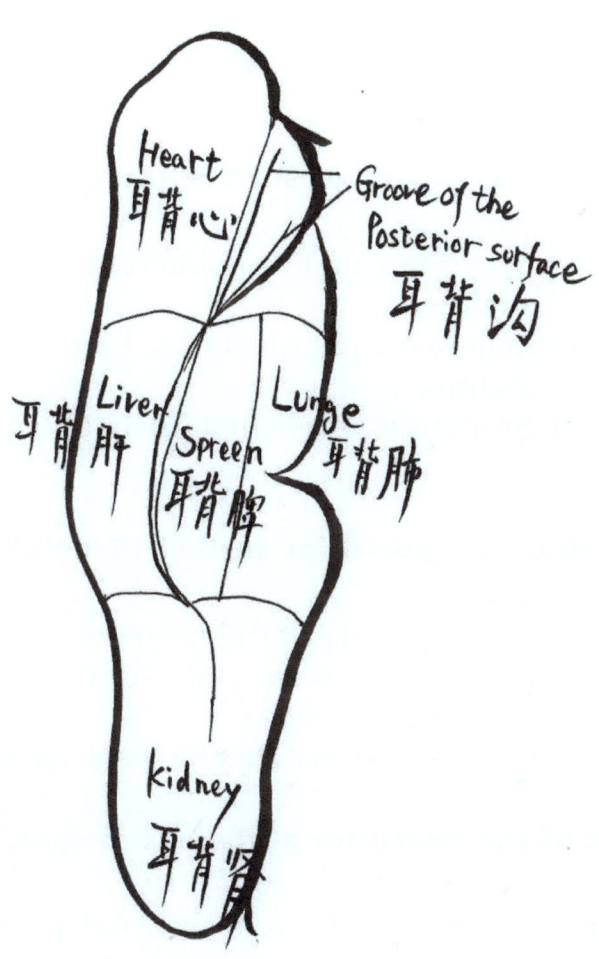

1. Heart of the posterior surface (Erbeixin 耳背心)

Location: On the superior, the posterior.
Function: Clear Heart heat, relieve mental stress.
Treatment: Hypertension,   palpitation,   insomnia,
            headache.

2. Lung of the posterior surface (Erbeifei 耳背肺)

Location: On   the   middle,   internal,   posterior.
            surface.
Function: Relieve cough, the flow of Lung Qi, relieve
            asthma.
Treatment: Bronchitis, bronchial asthma, cutaneous
            pruritus.

3. Spleen of the posterior surface (Erbeipi 耳背脾)

Location: On the center of the posterior surface.
Function: Regulate Spleen and Stomach, relieve
            pain and digestion.
Treatment: Gastritis, stomachache, poor appetite.

4. Liver of the posterior surface (Erbeigan 耳背肝)

Location: On the middle and external part of the
            posterior.

Function: Relieve Liver and Gallbladder, Qi circulation.

Treatment: Pain of hypochondriac region, cholecystitis.

5. Kidney of the posterior surface (Erbeishen 耳背肾)

Location: On the inferior part of the posterior.

Function: Nourish Liver and Kidney, strengthen bone and invigorate marrow, relieve spasm.

6. Groove of the posterior surface (Erbeigou 耳背沟)

Location: The groove formed by antihelix, superior, inferior antihelix, and on the posterior.

Function: Calm Liver, dispel wind, decrease blood pressure, relieve itching.

Treatment: Hypertension, headache.

10.Points on the Ear Root (Ergenxuewei 耳根穴位)

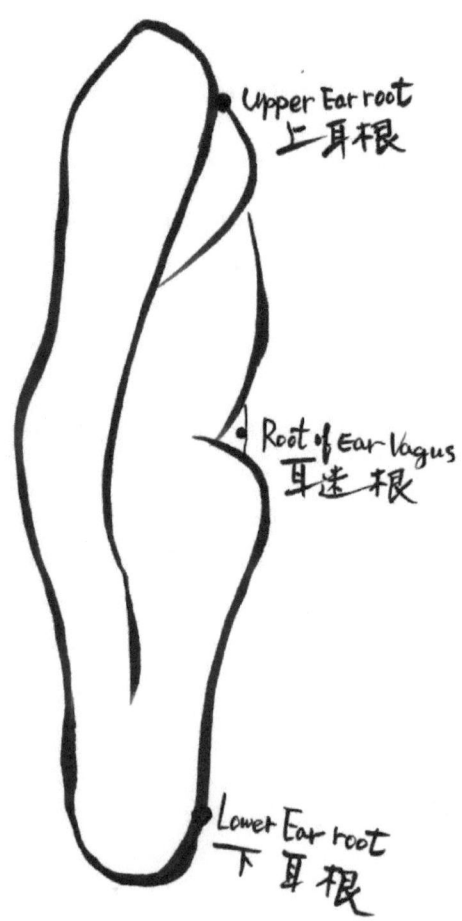

Upper Ear root
上耳根

Root of Ear Vagus
耳迷根

Lower Ear root
下耳根

1. Upper ear root (Shangergen 上耳根)

Location: On the uppermost part.
Function: Clear blood-heat.
Treatment:Epistaxis, paralysis.

2. Root of ear vagus (Ermigen 耳迷根)

Location: In the posterior groove formed by Helix.
Function: Clear heat and dampness, relieve spasm.
Treatment:Abdominal   pain,   diarrhea,   headache,
insomnia,   dizziness,   stomachache,
hypertension, retention of urine.

3. Lower ear root (Xiaergen 下耳根)

Location: On the lowest part.
Function: Nourish Liver and Kidney, relieve mental
stress.
Treatment:Hypotension, Bell's palsy.

IV. Clinical Application of Auricular Acupuncture

CHAPTER 1. Internal Diseases
Section 1. Circulatory and Respiratory
(1) Hypertension (Gaoxieya 高血压)

Main points
- Ear Apex (Erjian 耳尖)
- Wind stream (Fengxi 风溪)
- Superior triangular fossa (Jiaowoshang 角窝上)
- Shenmen (Shenmen 神门)
- Sympathesis (Jiaogan 交感)
- Heart (Xin 心)
- Subcortex (Pizhixia 皮质下)
- Groove of posterior surface (Erbeigou 耳背沟)

Secondary points
- Forehead (Zhen 枕)
- External ear (Waier 外耳)
- Kidney (Shen 肾)
- Hypertension point (Gaoxueyadian 高血压点)

(1) Hypertension (Gaoxieya 高血压)

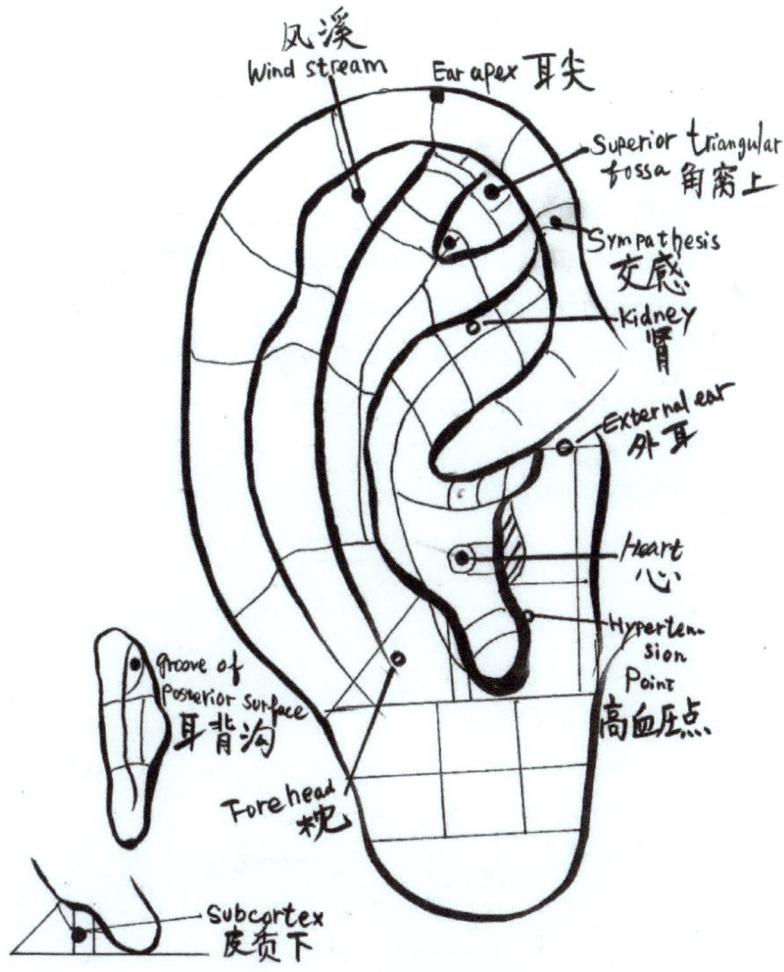

*Sympathesis (Jiaogan 交感) ⋯ covered

*Subcortex (Pizhixia 皮质下) ⋯ covered

(2) Hypotention (Dixieya 低血压)

Main points

- Heart (Xin 心)
- Adrenal gland (Shenshangxian 肾上腺)
- Central rim (Yuanzhong 缘中)
- Hypotension point (Dixueyadian 低血压点)
- Sympathesis (Jiaogan 交感)

Secondary points

- Subcortex (Pizhixia 皮质下)

(2) Hypotention (Dixieya 低血压)

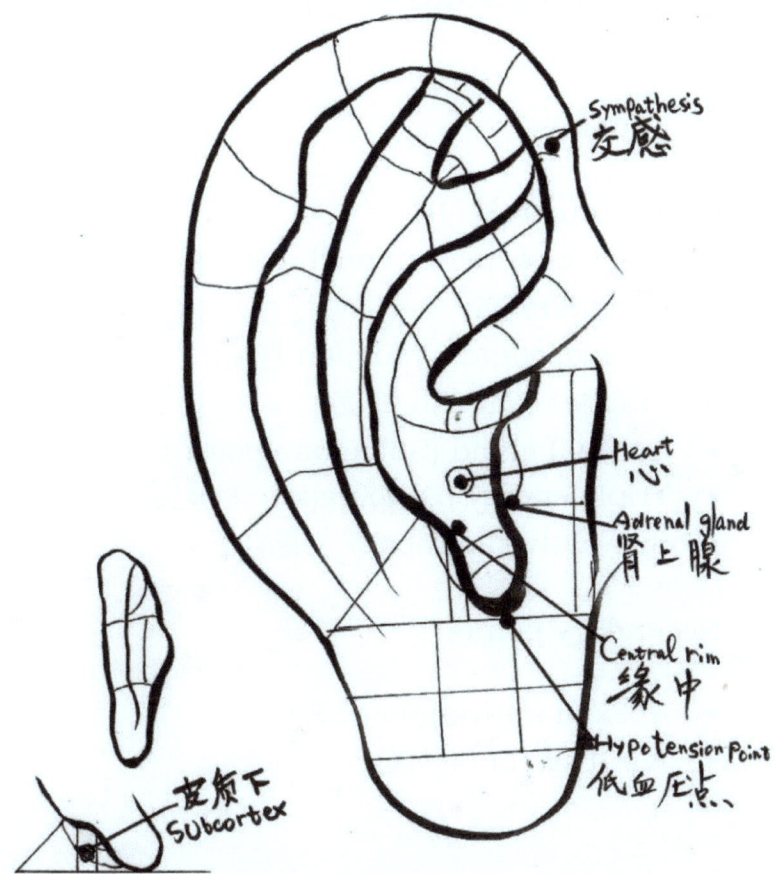

*Sympathesis (Jiaogan 交感) ⋯ covered

*Subcortex (Pizhixia 皮质下) ⋯ covered

(3) Bronchial Asthma (Zhiqiguanxiaochuan 支气管哮喘)

Main points

- Shenmen (神门)
- Angle of superior concha (Tingjiao 艇角)
- Lung (Fei 肺)
- Apex of tragus (Pingjian 屏尖)
- Trachea (Qiguan 气管)
- Adrenal gland (Shenshangxian 肾上腺)
- Triple energy (Duipingjian 对屏尖)
- Sympathesis (Jiaogan 交感)

Secondary points

- Apex of antitragus (三焦)
- Wind stream (风溪)

(3) Bronchial Asthma (Zhiqiguanxiaochuan 支气管哮喘)

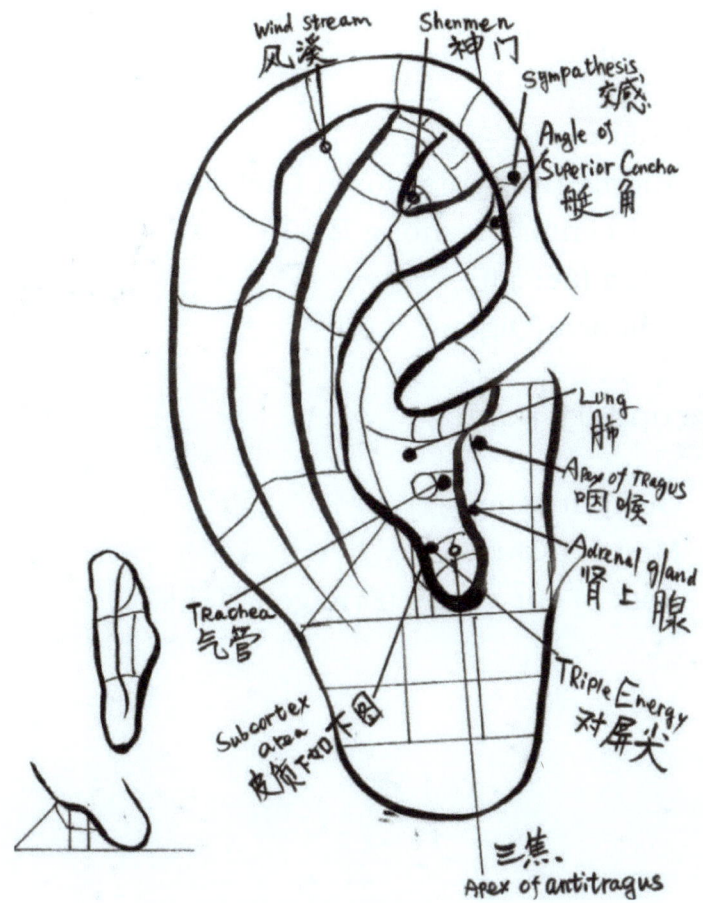

*Pharynx and larynx (Yanhou 咽喉)... covered
*Sympathesis (Jiaogan 交感)... covered

(4) Acute Bronchitis (Jixing zhiqiquanyan 急性支气管炎)

Main points

- Shenmen (神门)
- Middle triangular fossa (Jiaowozhong 角窝中)
- Ear center (Erzhong 耳中)
- Lung (Fei 肺)
- Trachea (Qiguan 气管)

Secondary points

- Occiput (Zhen 枕)
- Mouth (Kou 口)
- Root of ear vagus (Ermigen 耳迷根)

(4) Acute Bronchitis (Jixing zhiqiquanyan 急性支气管炎)

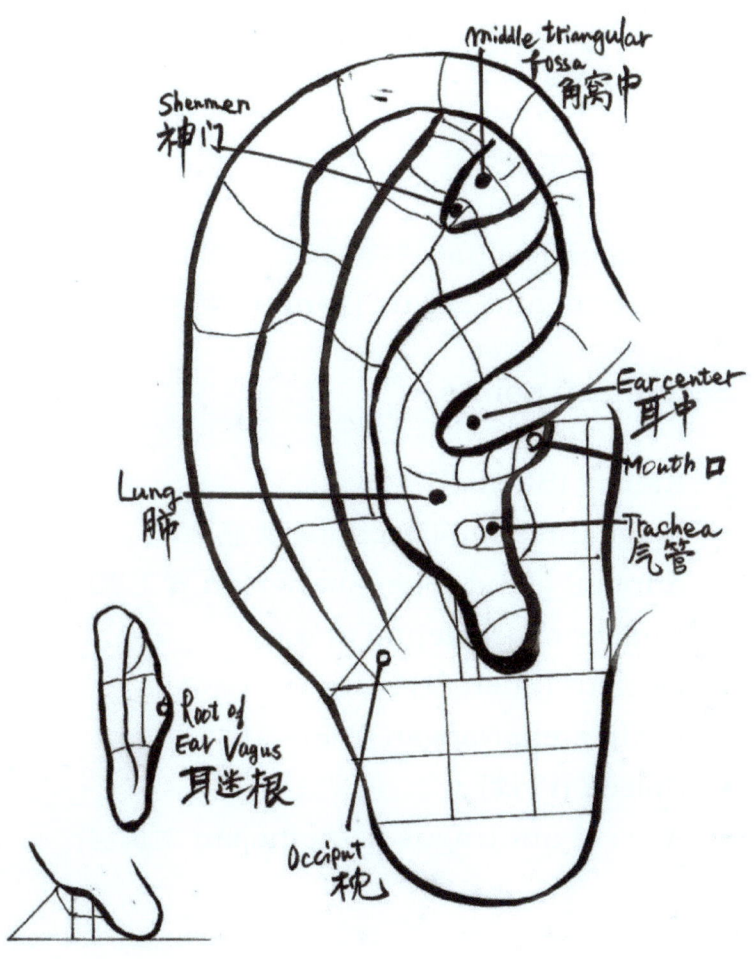

(5) Chronic Bronchitis (Manxing zhiqiguanyan 慢性支气管炎)

Main points

- Shenmen (神门)
- Lung (Fei 肺)
- Trachea (Qiguan 气管)
- Pharynx and larynx (Yanhou 咽喉)

Secondary points

- Kidney (Shen 肾)
- Large Intestine (Dachang 大肠)
- Adrenal gland (Shenshangxian 肾上腺)
- Endocrine (Neifenmi 内分泌)
- Occiput (Zhen 枕)
- Brain stem(Naogan 脑干)
- Spleen (Pi 脾)
- Apex of antitragus (Duipingjian 对屏尖)

(5) Chronic Bronchitis (Manxing zhiqiguanyan 慢性支气管炎)

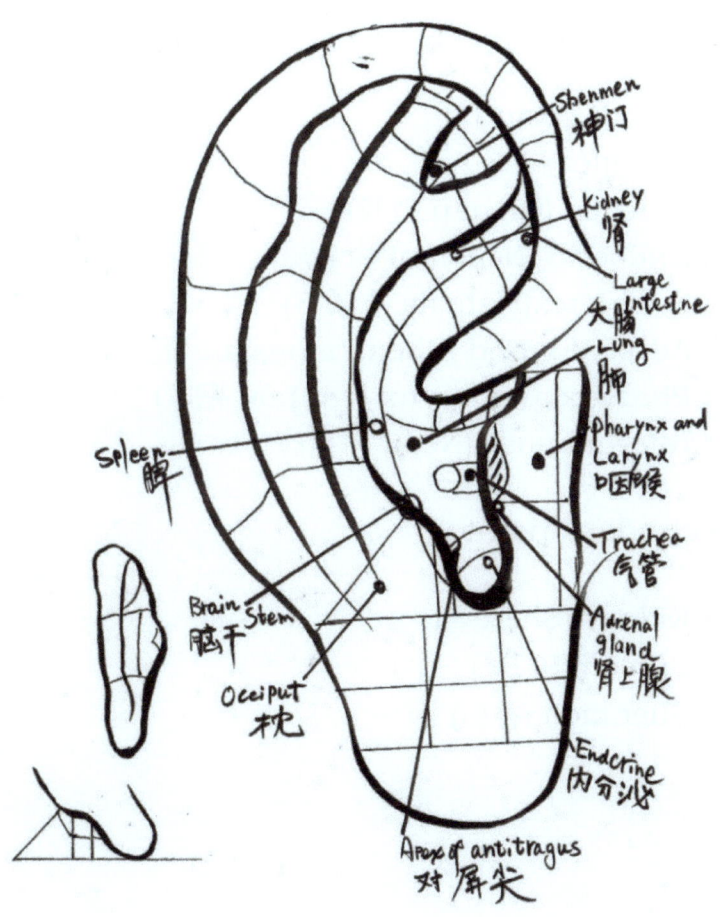

*Pharynx and larynx (Yanhou 咽喉)... covered

(6) Cough (Kesou 咳嗽)

Main points

- Mouth (Kou 口)
- Lung(fei 肺)
- Trachea (Qiguan 气管)
- Endocrin (Neifenmi 内分泌)
- Subcortex(Pizhixia 皮质下)
- Adrenal grand (Shenshangxian 肾上腺)
- Pharynx and larynx (Yanhou 咽喉)
- Internal nose (Neibi 内鼻)

Secondary points

- Kidney (Shen 肾)
- Spreen (Pi 脾)
- Shenmen (神门)

(6) Cough (Kesou 咳嗽)

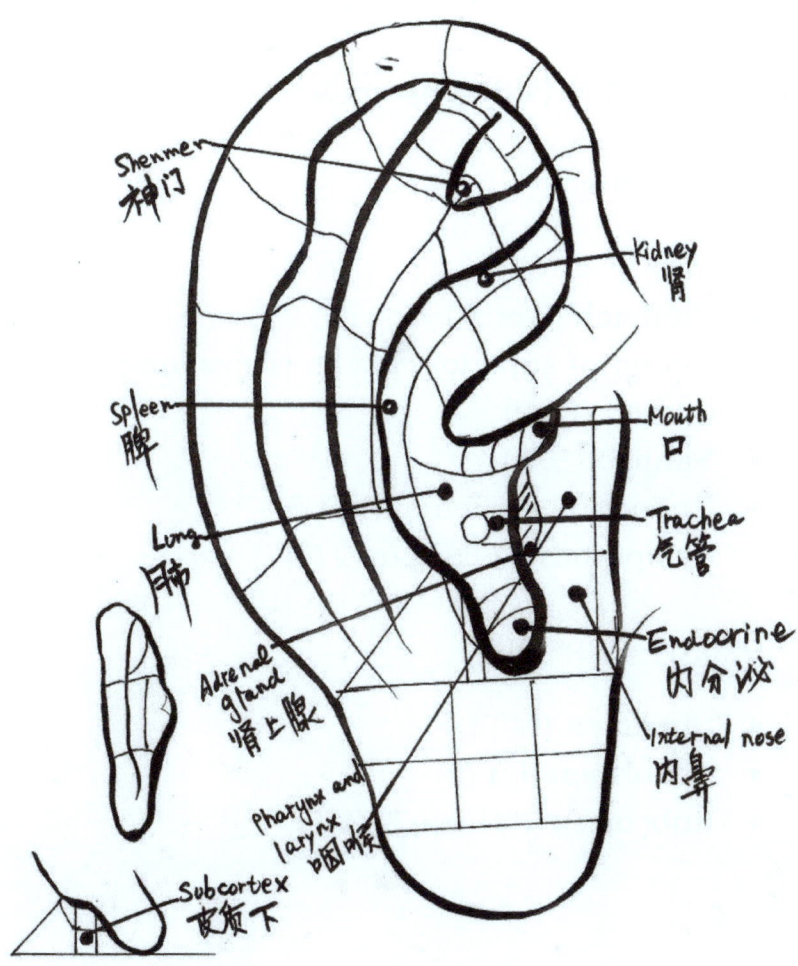

*Subcortex (Pizhixia 皮质下)⋯ covered

Section 2. Digestive System Disease

(1) Hepatitis (Ganyan 肝炎)

Main points

- Liver (Gan 肝)
- Stomach (Wei 胃)
- Center of superior concha (Tingzhong 艇中)
- Spreen (Pi 脾)
- Sanjiao (三焦)
- Endocrine (Neifenmi 内分泌)
- Sympathesis (Jiaogan 交感)

Secondary points

- Shenmen (神门)
- Abdormen (Fu 腹)
- Subcortex (Pizhixia 皮质下)

(1) Hepatitis (Ganyan 肝炎)

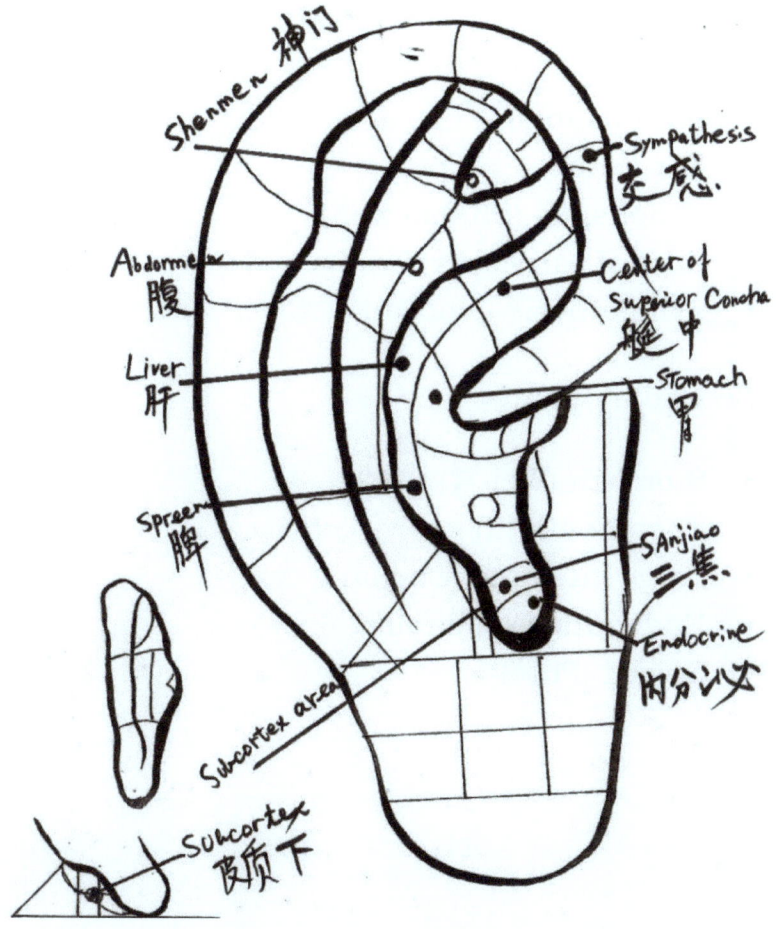

*Sympathesis (Jiaogan 交感)… covered
*Subcortex (Pizhixia 皮质下)… covered

(2) Hiccups (Eni 呃逆)

Main points

- Liver (Gan 肝)
- Ear center (Erzhong 耳中)
- Esophagus (Shidao 食道)
- Root of ear vagus (Ermigen 耳迷根)
- Sympathesis (Jiaogan 交感)

Secondary points

- Stomach (Wei 胃)
- Shenmen(神门)
- Large intestine (Dachang 大肠)
- Endocrine (Neifenmi 内分泌)
- Spleen (Pi 脾)

(2) Hiccups (Eni 呃逆)

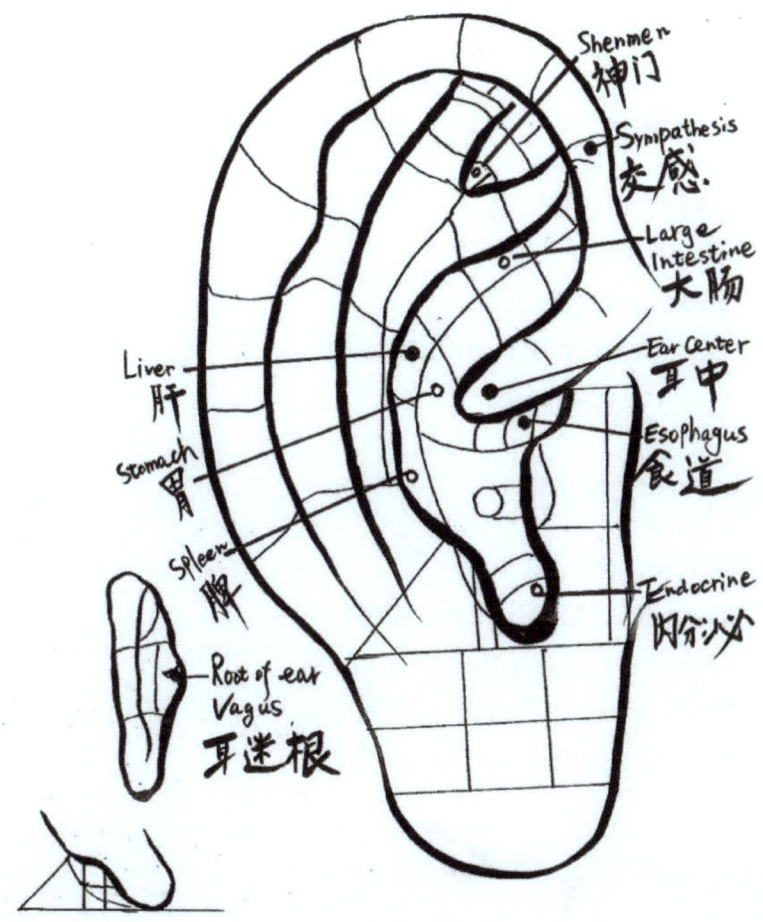

*Sympathesis (Jiaogan 交感)··· covered

(3) Nausea and Vomiting (Exinoutu 恶心 呕吐)

Main points

- Shenmen (神门)
- Liver (Gan 肝)
- Stomach (Wei 胃)
- Ear Center (Er zhong 耳中)
- Cardia (Benmen 贲门)

Secondary points

- Spleen (Pi 脾)
- Esophagus (Shidao 食道)
- Sympathesis (Jiaogan 交感)
- Subcortex (Pizhixia 皮质下)
- Endocrine (Neifenbi 内分泌)

(3) Nausea and Vomiting (Exinoutu 恶心 呕吐)

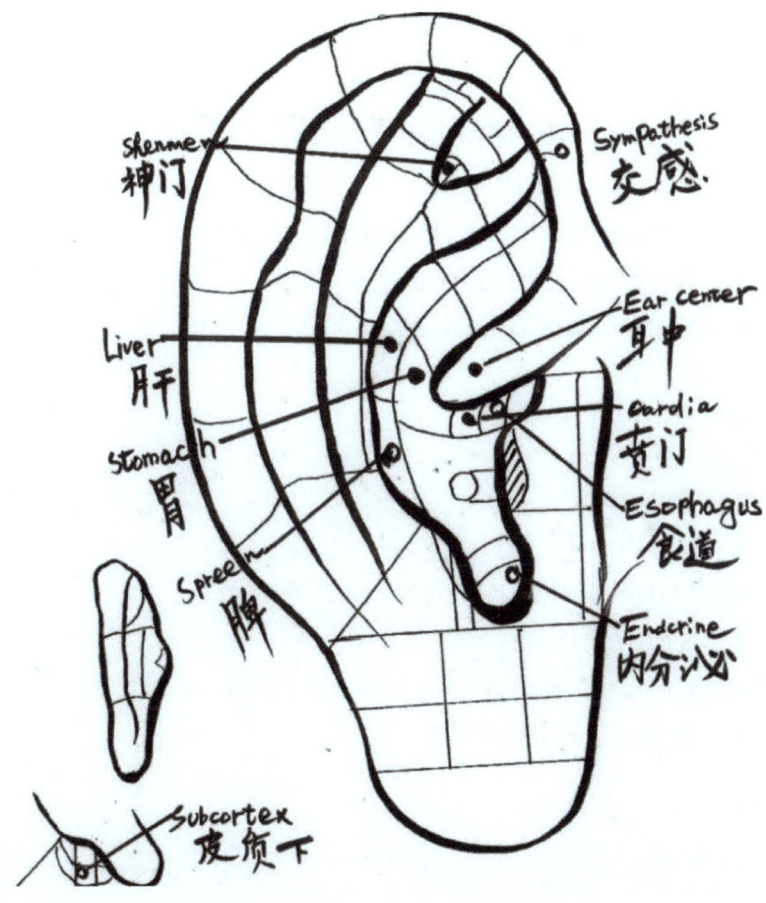

*Sympathesis (Jiaogan 交感)··· covered
*Subcortex (Pizhixia 皮质下)··· covered

(4) Constipation (Bianmi 便秘)

Main points

- Constipation point (Bianmidian 便秘点)
- Abdormen (Fu 腹)
- Large Intestine (Dachang 大肠)
- Rectum (Zhichang 直肠)
- Subcortex (Pizhixia 皮质下)

Secondary points

- Sanjiao (三焦)
- Spreen(Pi 脾)
- Lung (Fei 肺)
- Kidney (Shen 肾)
- Heart (Xin 心)
- Stomach (Wei 胃)

(4) Constipation (Bianmi 便秘)

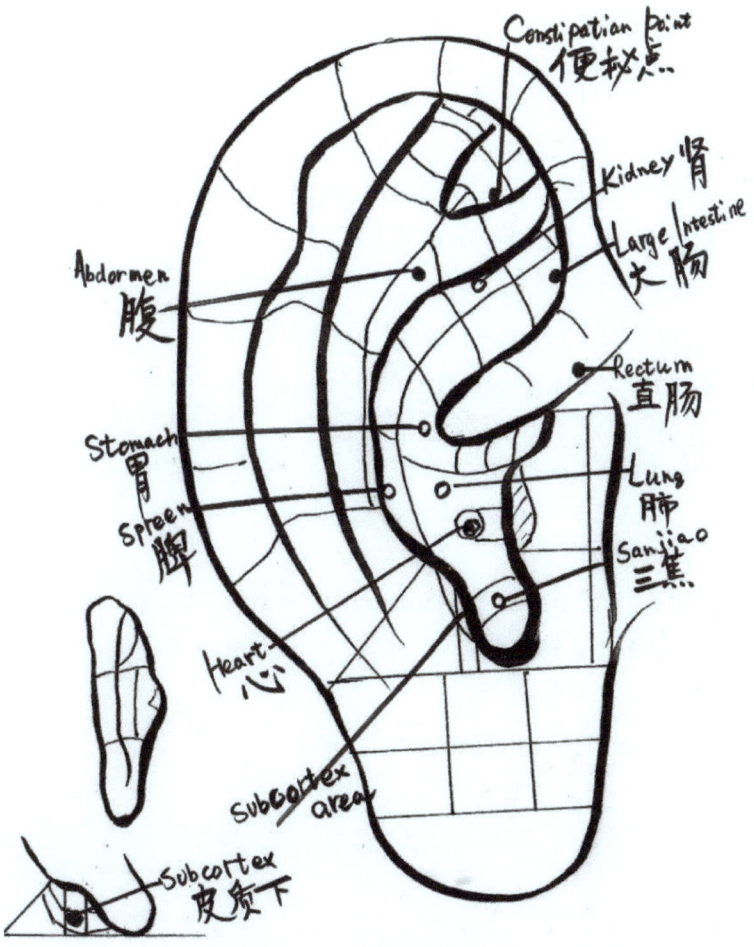

*Subcortex (Pizhixia 皮质下)… covered

(5) Diarrhea (Fuxie 腹泻)

Main points

- Shenmen (神门)
- Abdomen (Fu 腹)
- Large Intestine (Dachang 大肠)
- Rectum (Zhichang 直肠)
- Stomach (Wei 胃)
- Apex of Tragus (Pingjian 屏尖)
- Endocrine (Neifenmi 内分泌)

Secondary points

- Spleen (Pi 脾)
- Small Intestine (Xiaochan 小肠)
- Sanjao(三焦)
- Kidney (Shen 肾)
- Sympathesis(Jiaogan 交感)

(5) Diarrhea (Fuxie 腹泻)

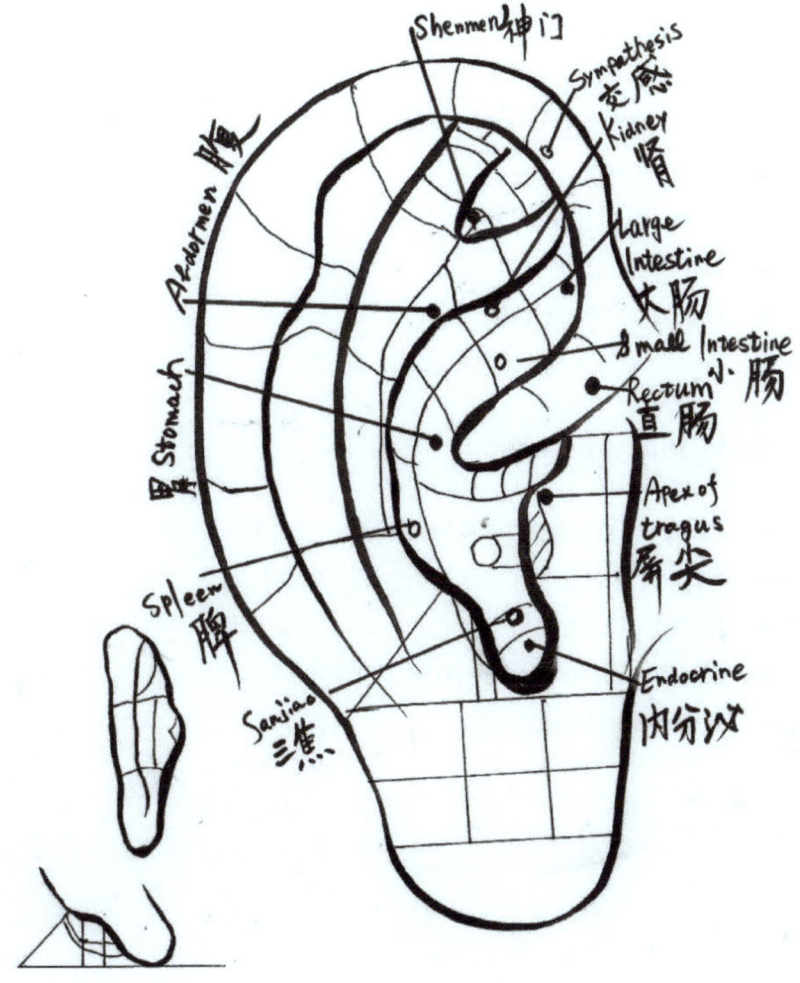

*Sympathesis (Jiaogan 交感)⋯ covered

(6) Gastritis (Weiyan 胃炎)

Main points

- Ear apex (Erjian 耳尖)
- Shenmen (神门)
- Stomach(Wei 胃)
- Lung (Fei 肺)
- Subcortex (皮质下))
- Sympathesis (Jiaogan 交感)

Secondary points

- Large Intestine (Dachang 大肠)
- Spreen (Pi 脾)
- Liver (Gan 肝)
- Endocrine (Neifenmi 内分泌)
- Kidney (Shen 肾)

(6) Gastritis (Weiyan 胃炎)

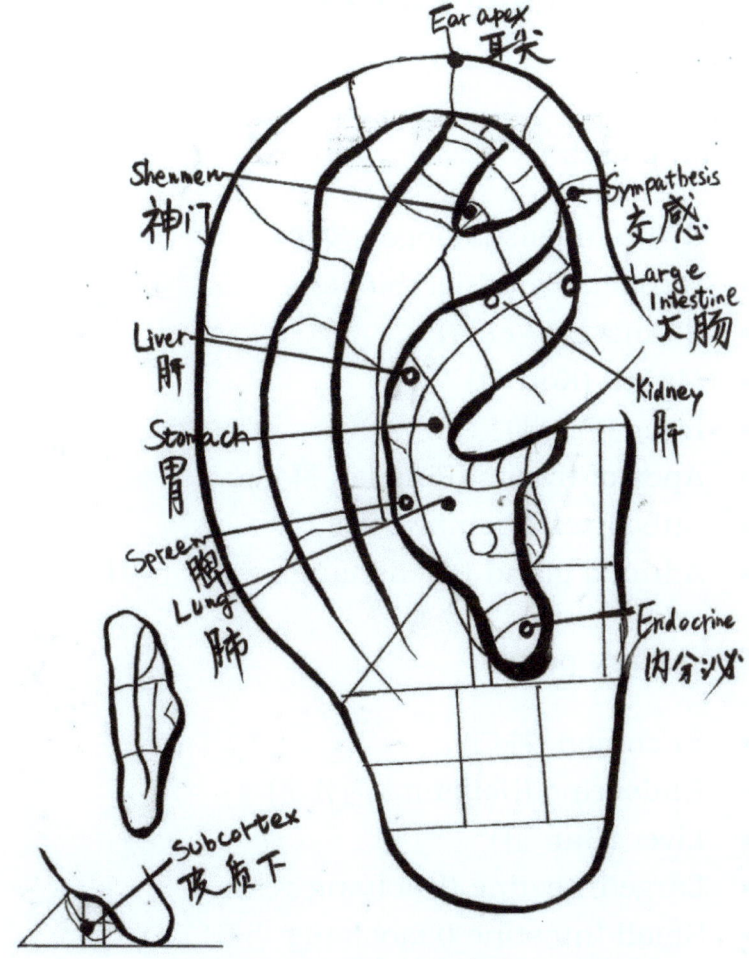

*Sympathesis (Jiaogan 交感)⋯ covered
*Subcortex (Pizhixia 皮质下)⋯ covered

(7) Gastritis and Duodenal Ulcer (Weiyan he shierzhichang kuiyang 胃，十二指肠肠溃疡)

Main points

- Sympathesis (Jiaogan 交感)
- Duodenum (Shierzhichang 十二指肠)
- Stomach (Wei 胃)
- Mouth (Kou 口)
- Lung (Fei 肺)
- Apex of tragus (Pingjian 屏尖)
- Subcortex (Pizhixia 皮质下)
- Adrenal gland (shenshangxian 肾上腺)

Secondary points

- Shenmen (神门)
- Endocrine (Neifenmi 内分泌)
- Liver (Gan 肝)
- Large Intestine (Dachang 大肠)
- Small Intestine (xiaochang 小肠)
- Spleen (Pi 脾)

(7) Gastritis and Duodenal Ulcer (Weiyan he shierzhichang kuiyang 胃，十二指肠肠溃疡)

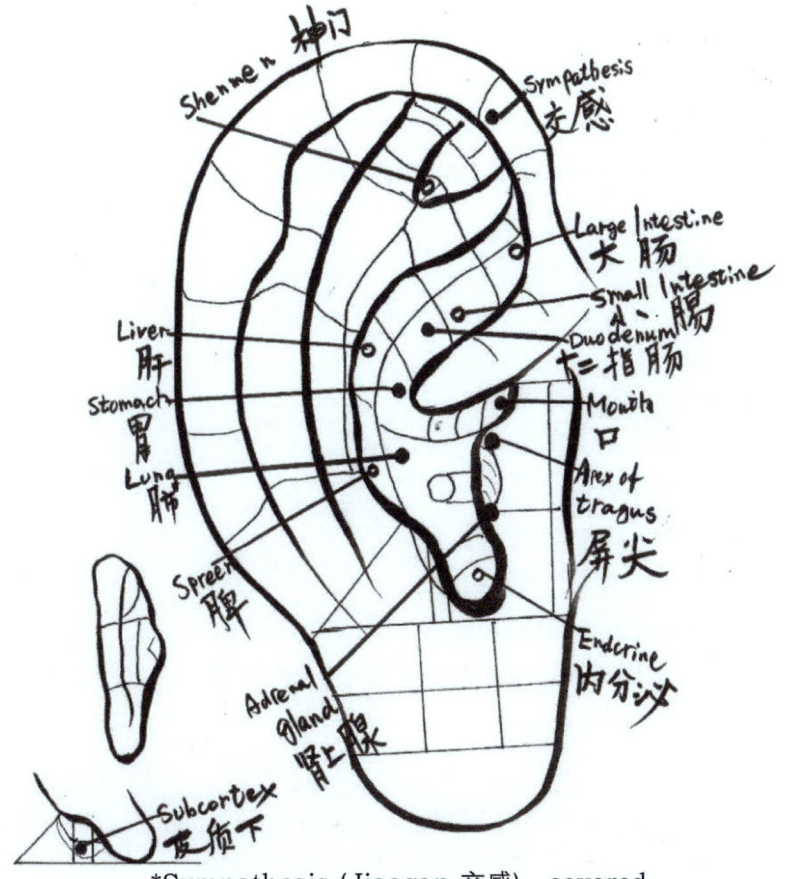

*Sympathesis (Jiaogan 交感)··· covered
*Subcortex (Pizhixia 皮质下)··· covered

(8) Chronic Cholecystitis (Manxing dannangyan 慢性胆囊炎)

Main points

- Sympathesis (Jiaogan 交感)
- Pancreas and gallbladder (胰胆)
- Liver (Gan 肝)
- Mouth (Kou 口)
- Endocrine (Neifenmi 内分泌)

Secondary points

- Sanjiao (三焦)
- Shenmen (神门)
- Spleen (Pi 脾)
- Stomach (Wei 胃)
- Root of ear vagus (Ermigen 耳迷根)

(8) Chronic Cholecystitis (Manxing dannangyan 慢性胆囊炎)

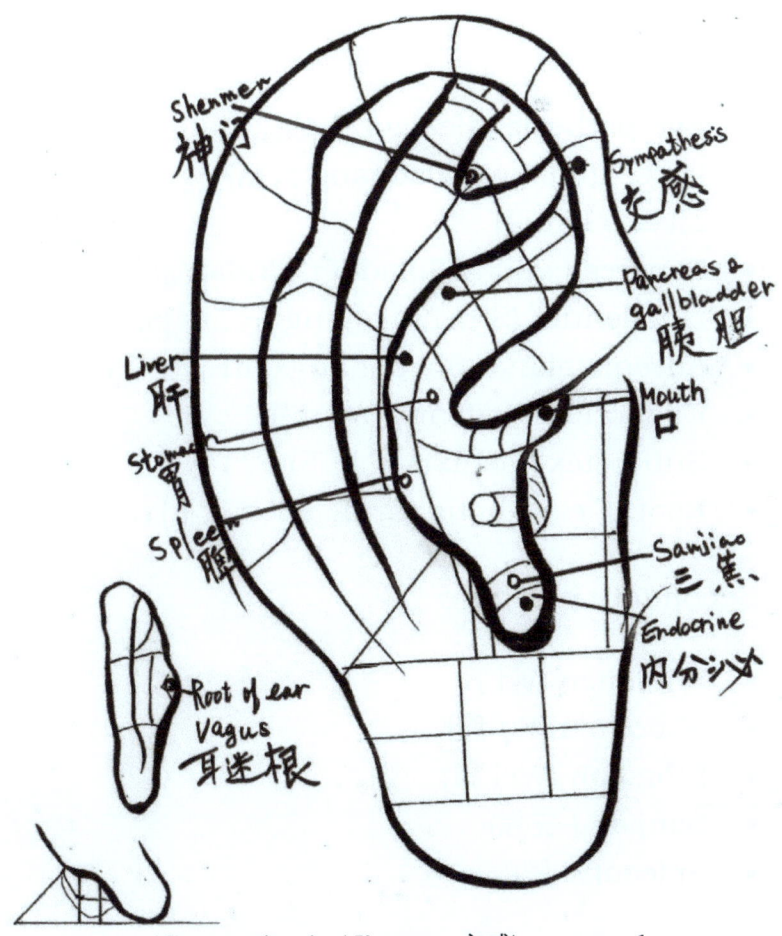

*Sympathesis (Jiaogan 交感)··· covered

(9) Cholelithiasis, Gallstone (Danshizheng 胆石症)

Main points

- Sympathesis (Jiaogan 交感)
- Large Intestine (Dachang 大肠)
- Liver (Gan 肝)
- Pancreas and gallbladder (Yidan 胰胆)
- Duodenum (Shierzhichang 十二指肠)
- Adrenal gland (Shenshangxian 肾上腺)
- Endocrine (Neifenmi 内分泌)
- Subcortex (Pizhixia 皮质下)
- Root of ear Vagus (Ermigen 耳迷根)

Secondary points

- Shenmen (神门)
- Abdomen (Fu 腹)
- Stomach (Wei 胃)
- Sanjiao (三焦)
- Spleen(Pi 脾)

(9) Cholelithiasis, Gallstone (Danshizheng 胆石症)

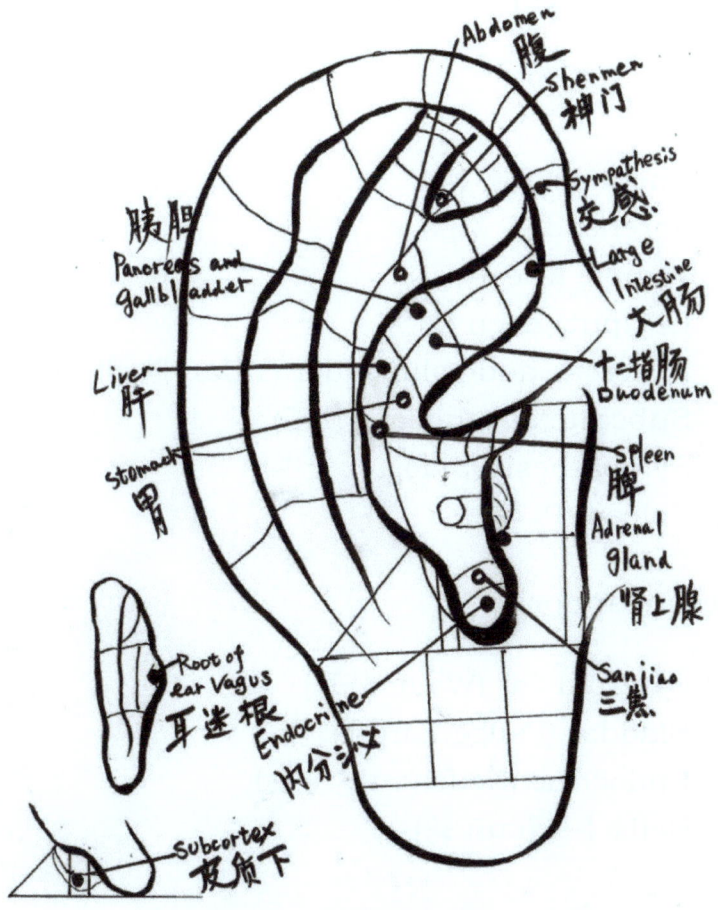

*Sympathesis (Jiaogan 交感)… covered
*Subcortex (Pizhixia 皮质下)… covered

Section 3. Neurotic and Mental Diseases

(1) Headache (Toutong 头痛)

Main points

- Shenmen (神门)
- Forehead (E 额)
- Temple (Nie 颞)
- Occiput (Zhen 枕)
- Pancreas and gallbladder (Yidan 胰胆)
- Subcortex (Pizhixia 皮质下)
- Sympathesis (Jiaogan 交感)
- Spleen (Pi 脾)

Secondary points

- External ear (Waier 外耳)
- Bladder (Pangguang 膀胱)
- Endocrine (Neifenmi 内分泌)
- Helix 1-4 (Lun 轮)

(1) Headache (Toutong 头痛)

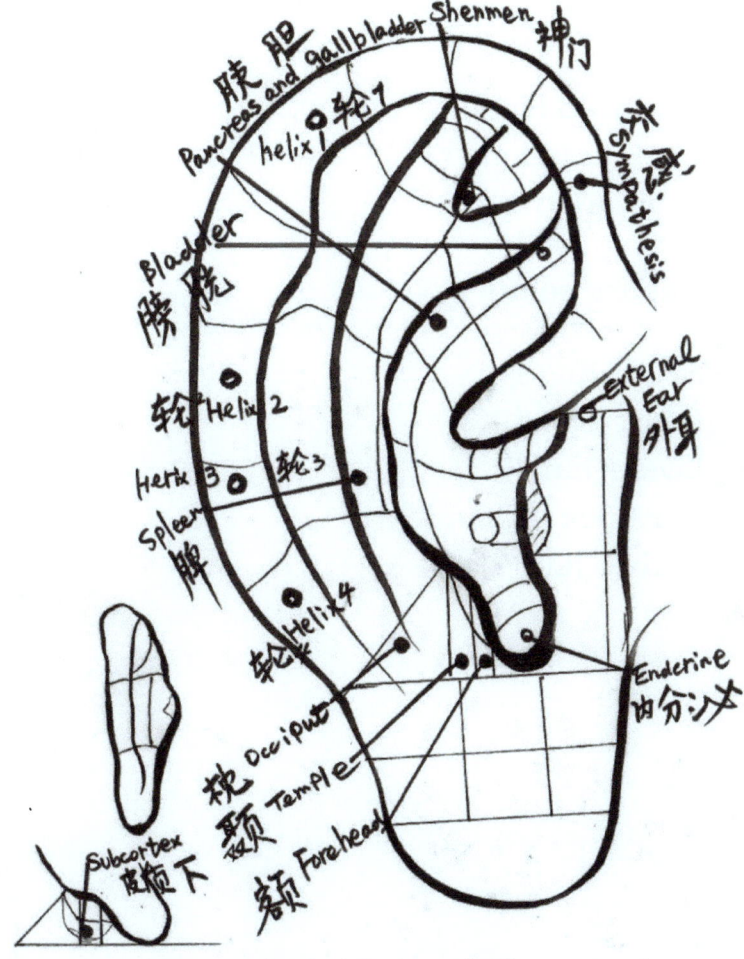

*Sympathesis (Jiaogan 交感)··· covered
*Subcortex (Pizhixia 皮质下)... covered

(2) Migraine (Piantoutong 偏头痛)

Main points

- Forehead (E 额)
- Occiput (Zhen 枕)
- Brain (Nao 脑)

Secondary points

- Neck (Jing 颈)
- Heart (Xin 心)
- Liver (Gan 肝)
- Ear Apex (Erjian 耳尖)
- Helix 6 (Lun 轮)

(2) Migraine (Piantoutong 偏头痛)

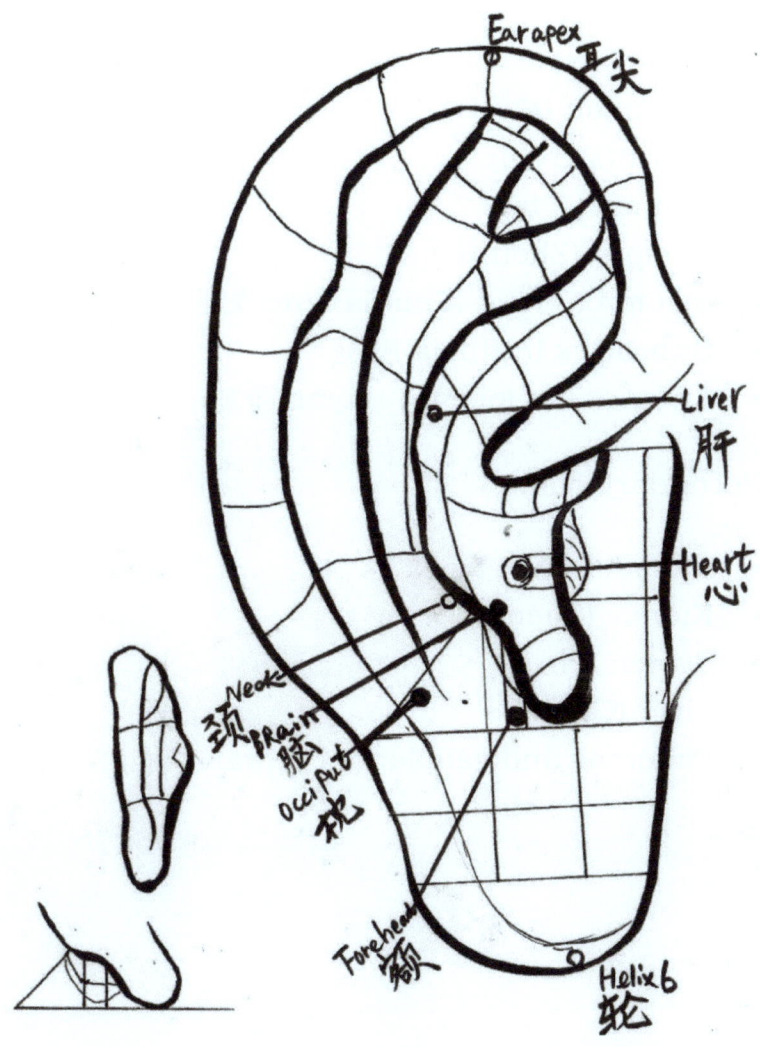

(3) Insomnia (Shimian 失眠)

Main Points

- Shenmen (神门)
- Heart (Xin 心)
- Sanjiao (三焦)
- Occiput (Zhen 枕)
- Insomnia point (Shimianxue 失眠穴)
- Subcortex (Pizhixia 皮质下)
- Anterior ear lobe (Chuiqian 垂前)

Secondary points

- Stomach (Wei 胃)
- Kidney (Shen 肾)
- Spleen (Pi 脾)
- Liver (Gan 肝)
- Pancreas and gallbladder (Yidan 胰胆)

(3)Insomnia (Shimian 失眠)

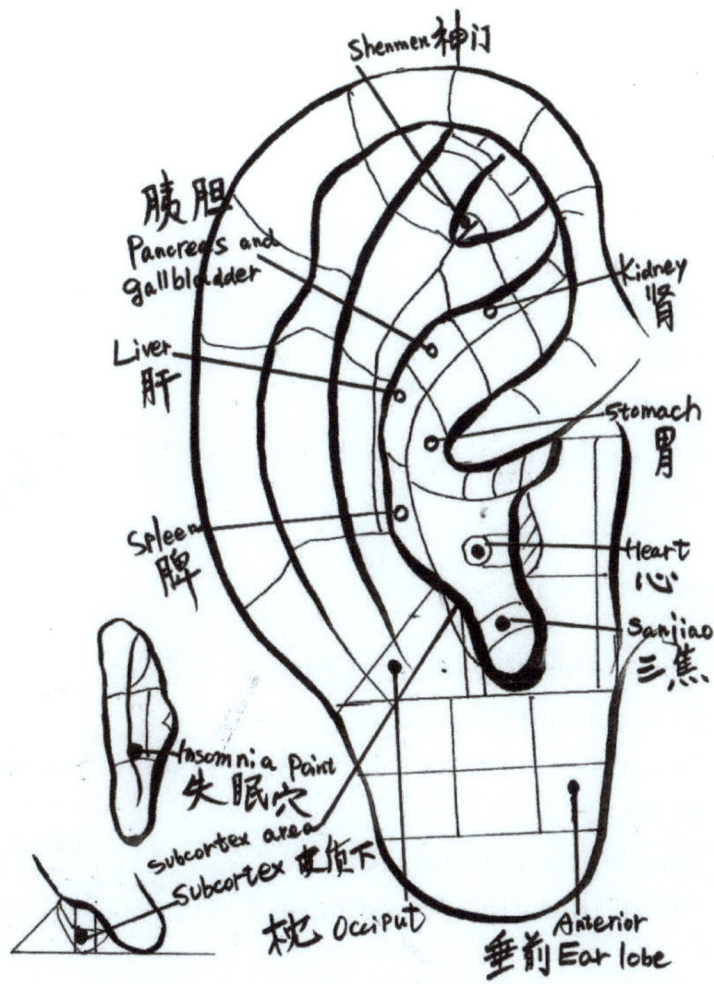

Shenmen 神门

胰胆
Pancreas and gallbladder

Kidney 肾

Liver 肝

Stomach 胃

Spleen 脾

Heart 心

Sanjiao 三焦

Insomnia Point 失眠穴

Subcortex area
Subcortex 皮质下

枕 Occiput

垂前 Anterior Ear lobe

*Subcortex (Pizhixia 皮质下)⋯ covered

(4) Epilepsy (Dianxian 癫痫)

Main points

- Shenmen (神门)
- Kidney (Shen 肾)
- Liver (Gan 肝)
- Stomach (Wei 胃)
- Spleen (Pi 脾)
- Heart (Xin 心)
- Sanjiao (三焦)
- Occiput (Zhen 枕)
- Subcortex (Pizhixia 皮质下)

Secondary points

- Brain stem (Naogan 脑干)
- Central rim (Yuanzhong 缘中)
- Nervus occipitalis minor (Zhenxiaoshenjing 枕小神经)
- Ear center (Erzhong 耳中)
- Small intestine (Xiaochang 小肠)

(4)Epilepsy (Dianxian 癲癇)

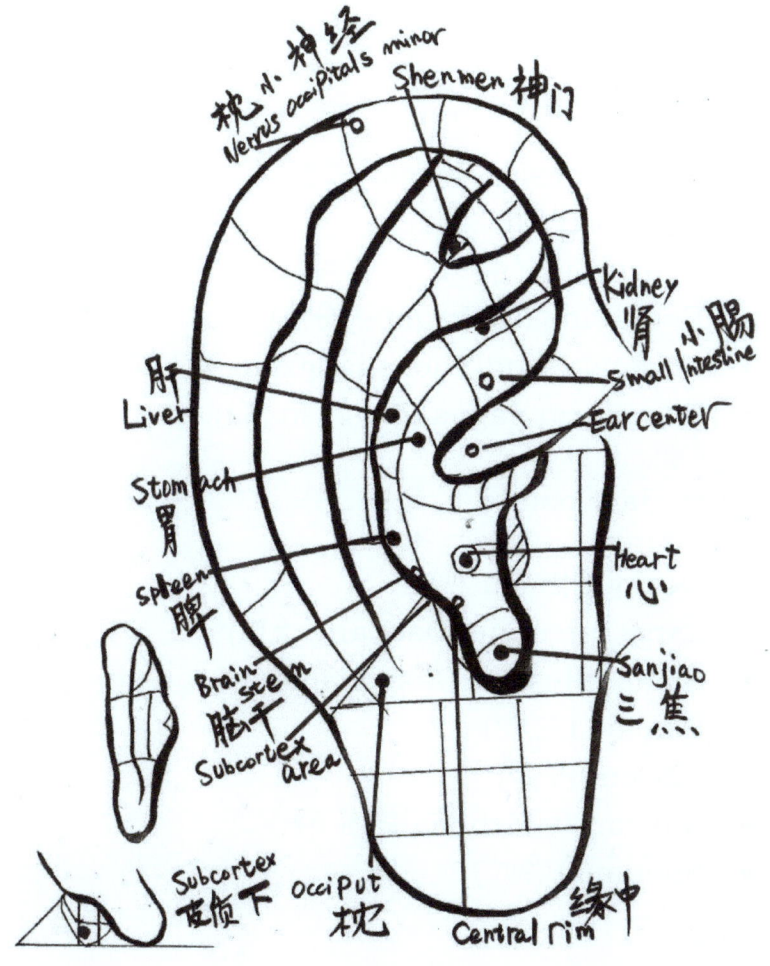

*Subcortex (Pizhixia 皮质下)… covered

(5) Hyperhidrosis (Duohanzheng 多汗症)

Main points

- Sympathesis (Jiaogan 交感)
- Lung (Fei 肺)
- Heart (Xin 心)
- Endocrine (Neifenmi 内分泌)
- Adrenal gland(Shenshangxian 肾上腺)
- Root of ear vagus (Ermigen 耳迷根)

Secondary points

- Occiput (Zhen 枕)
- Large intestine (Dachang 大肠)
- Small intestine (Xiaochang 小肠)
- Sanjiao (三焦)
- Spleen (Pi 脾)
- Subcortex(Pizhixia 皮质下)
- Shenmen (神门)

(5)Hyperhidrosis (Duohanzheng 多汗症)

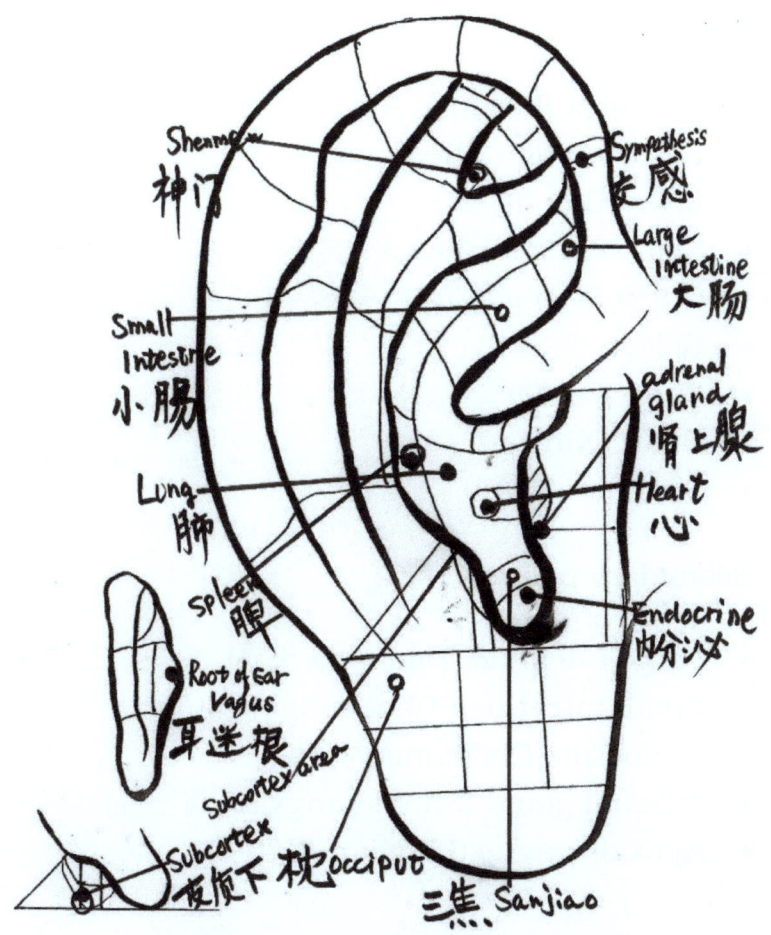

*Sympathesis (Jiaogan 交感)… covered
*Subcortex (Pizhixia 皮质下)… covered

(6) Chest Pain (Xiongtong 胸痛)

Main points

- Ear apex (Erjian 耳尖)
- Kidney (Shen 肾)
- Liver (Gan 肝)
- Sympathesis (Jiaogan 交感)
- Chest (Xiong 胸)
- Spleen (Pi 脾)
- Lung (Fei 肺)
- Heart (Xin 心)
- Shenmen (神门)

Secondary points

- Large intestine (Dachang 大肠)
- Small intestine (Xiaochang 小肠)
- Endocrine (Neifenmi 内分泌)
- Adrenal gland (Shenshangxian 肾上腺)
- Apex of tragus (Pingjian 屏尖)

(6)Chest Pain (Xiongtong 胸痛)

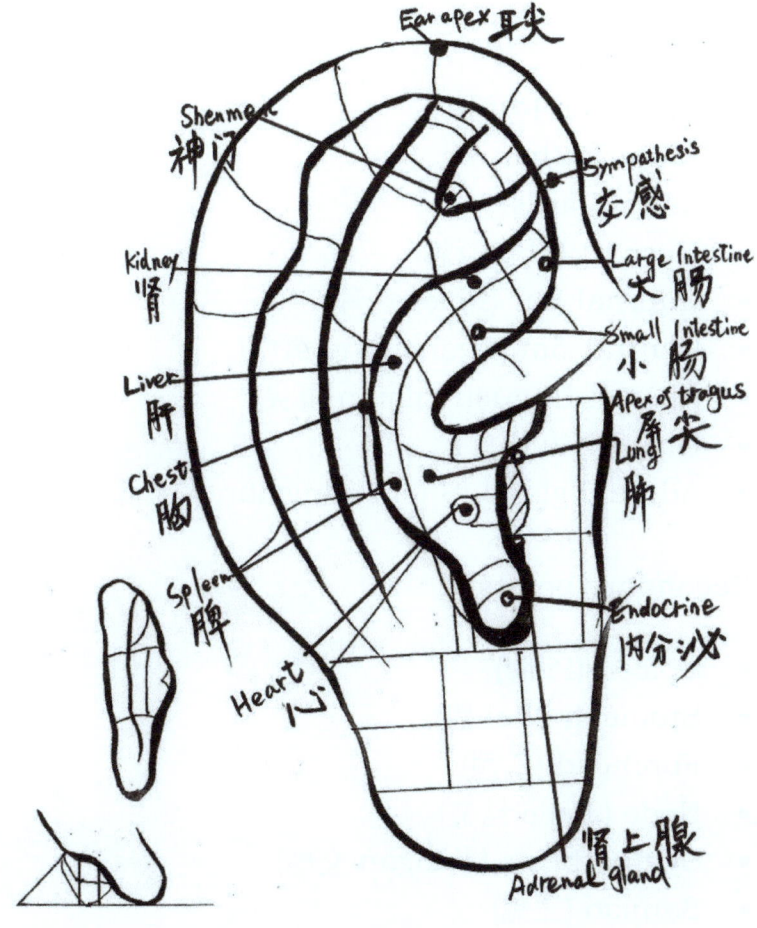

Ear apex 耳尖
Shenmen 神门
Sympathesis 交感
Kidney 肾
Large Intestine 大肠
Small Intestine 小肠
Liver 肝
Apex of tragus 屏尖
Lung 肺
Chest 胸
Spleen 脾
Endocrine 内分泌
Heart 心
肾上腺 Adrenal gland

*Sympathesis (Jiaogan 交感)… covered

(7) Vertigo, Dizzy (Xuan yun 眩晕)

Main points

- Shenmen (神门)
- Kidney (Shen 肾)
- Liver (Gan 肝)
- Occiput (Zhen 枕)
- Internal Ear (Neier 内耳)
- Central rim (Yuanzhong 缘中)
- Apex of tragus(Pingjian 屏尖)
- Heart (Xin 心)
- Adrenal gland (Shenshangxian 肾上腺)

Secondary points

- Spleen (Pi 脾)
- Stomach (Wei 胃)
- Forehead (E 额)
- Node (Jiejie 结节)
- Sympathesis (Jiaogan 交感)
- Sanjiao (三焦)
- Endocrine (Neifenmi 内分泌)

(7)Vertigo, Dizzy (Xuan yun 眩晕)

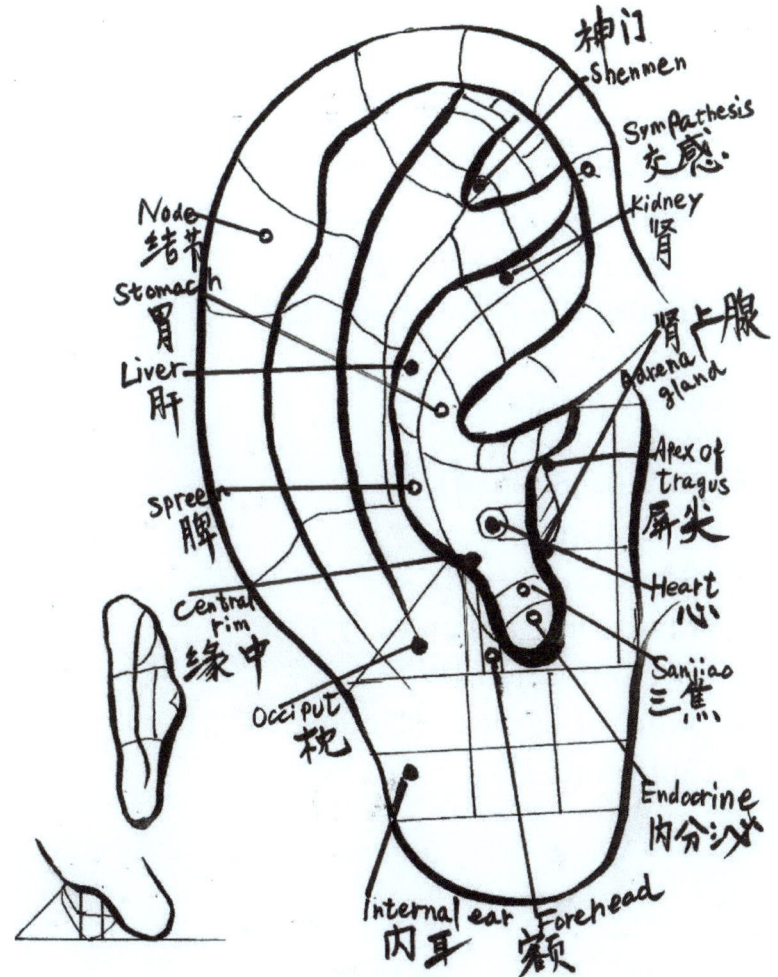

神门
Shenmen

Sympathesis
交感.

Kidney
肾

肾上腺
Adrenal
gland

Apex of
tragus
屏尖

Heart
心

Sanjiao
三焦

Endocrine
内分泌

Node
结带

Stomach
胃

Liver
肝

Spreen
脾

Central
rim
缘中

Occiput
枕

Internal ear
内耳

Forehead
额

*Sympathesis (Jiaogan 交感)… covered

(8) Neurosism (Shenjingshuairuo 神经衰弱)

Main points

- Shenmen (神门)
- Ear center (Erzhong 耳中)
- Heart (Xin 心)
- Subcortex (Pizhixia 皮质下)
- Central rim (Yuanzhong 缘中)

Secodary points

- Kidney (Shen 肾)
- Liver (Gan 肝)
- Stomach (Wei 胃)
- Endocrine (Neifenmi 内分泌)
- Occiput (Zhen 枕)
- Anterior ear lobe (Chuiqian 垂前)
- Spleen (Pi 脾)

(8)Neurosism (Shenjingshuairuo 神经衰弱)

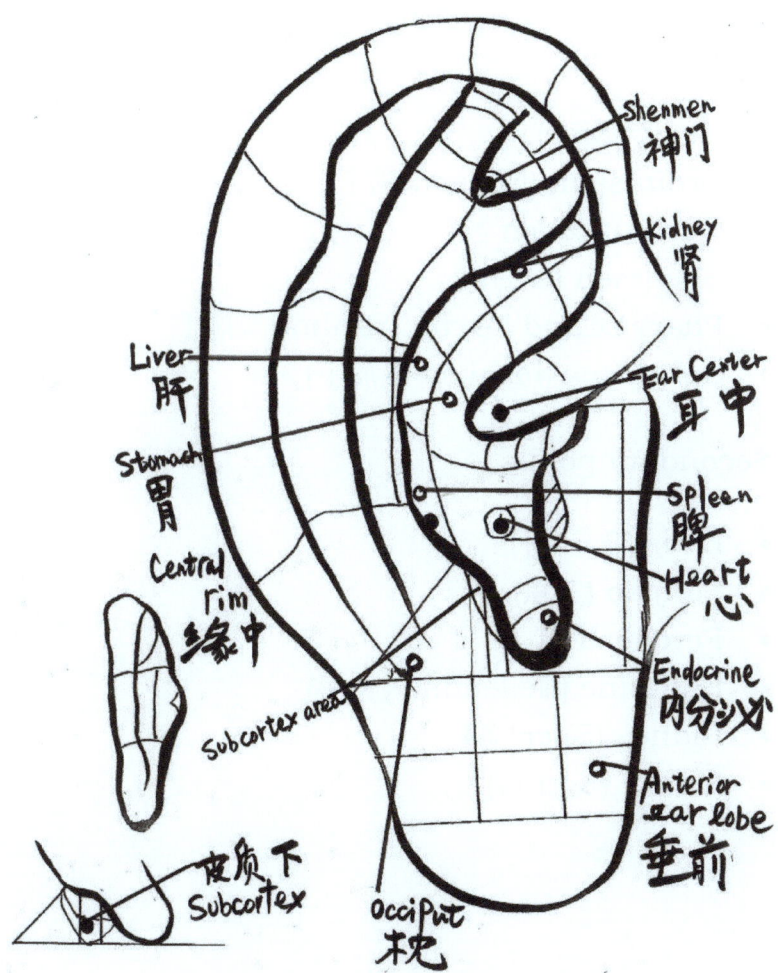

Shenmen 神门

Kidney 肾

Liver 肝

Ear Center 耳中

Stomach 胃

Spleen 脾

Heart 心

Central rim 缘中

Endocrine 内分泌

Subcortex area

Anterior ear lobe 垂前

皮质下 Subcortex

Occiput 枕

*Subcortex (Pizhixia 皮质下)… covered

(9) Hysteria (Xiesidili 歇斯底里)

Main points

- Heart (Xin 心)
- Brain stem (Naogan 脑干)
- Occiput (Zhen 枕)
- Shenmen (神门)
- Pharynx and larynx (Yanhou 咽喉)
- Subcortex (Pizhixia 皮质下)

Secondary points

- Liver (Gan 肝)
- Sanjiao (三焦)
- Forehead (E 额)
- Endcrine (Neifenmi 内分泌)
- Kidney (Shen 肾)
- Mouth (Kou 口)

(9) Hysteria (Xiesidili 歇斯底里)

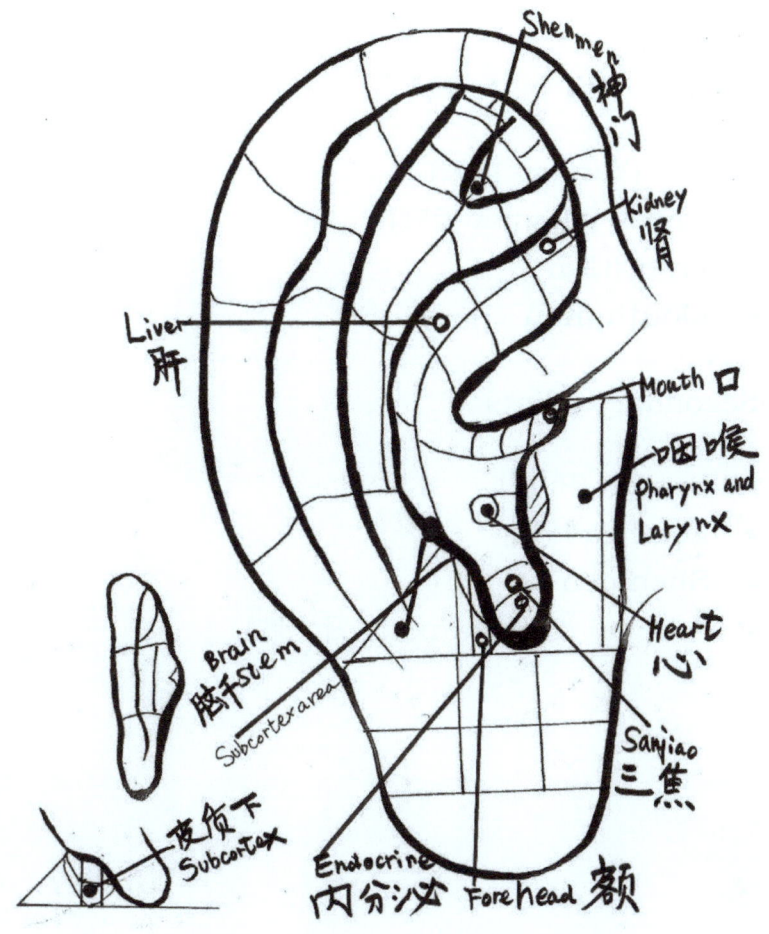

*Subcortex (Pizhixia 皮质下)… covered
*Pharynx and larynx (Yanhou 咽喉) covered

(10) Facial Neuritis (Mianshenjingyan 面神经炎)

Main points

- Eye (Yanjing 眼睛)
- Cheek (Mianjia 面颊)
- Liver (Gan 肝)
- Mouth (Kou 口)

Secondary points

- Spreen (Pi 脾)
- Forehead (额)
- Shenmen (神门)
- Adrenal (Senshanxian 肾上腺)

(10) Facial Neuritis (Mianshenjingyan 面神经炎)

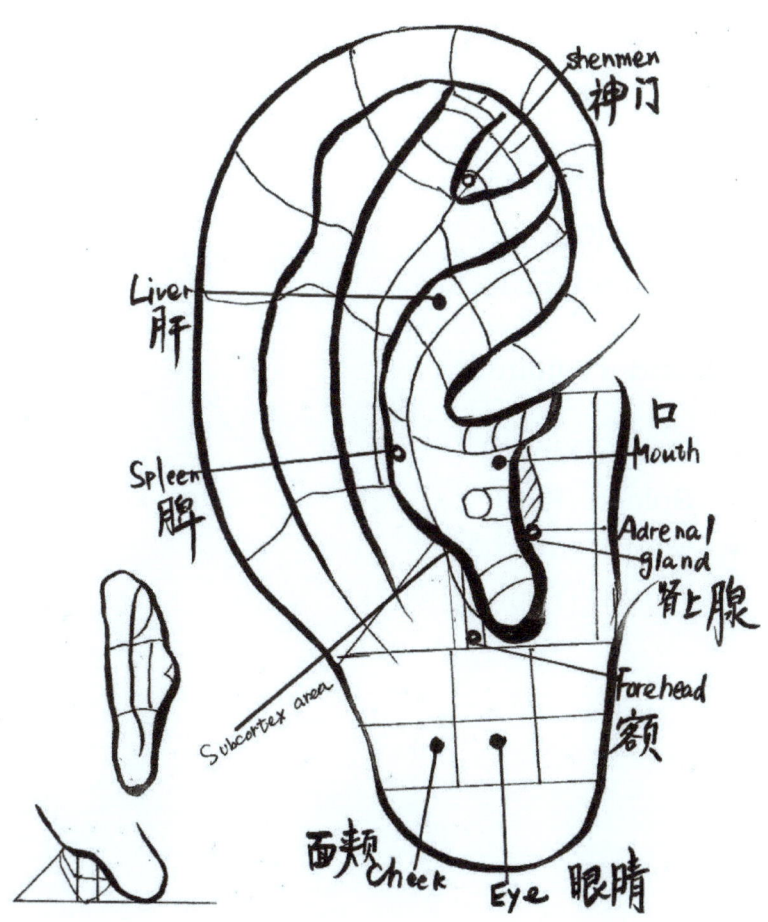

shenmen 神门

Liver 肝

Spleen 脾

口 Mouth

Adrenal gland 肾上腺

Forehead 额

Subcortex area

面颊 Cheek   Eye 眼睛

(11) Sequelae of Cerebrovascular Accident (Naoxieguanywaihoouyizheng 脑血棺意外后遗症)

Main points

- Brain (Nao 脑)
- Liver (Gan 肝)
- Sanjiao (三焦)

Secondary points

- Heart (Xin 心)
- Spleen (Pi 脾)
- Mouth (Kou 口)
- Throat (Yanhou 咽喉)

(11) Sequelae of Cerebrovascular Accident (Naoxieguanywaihoouyizheng 脑血棺意外后遗症)

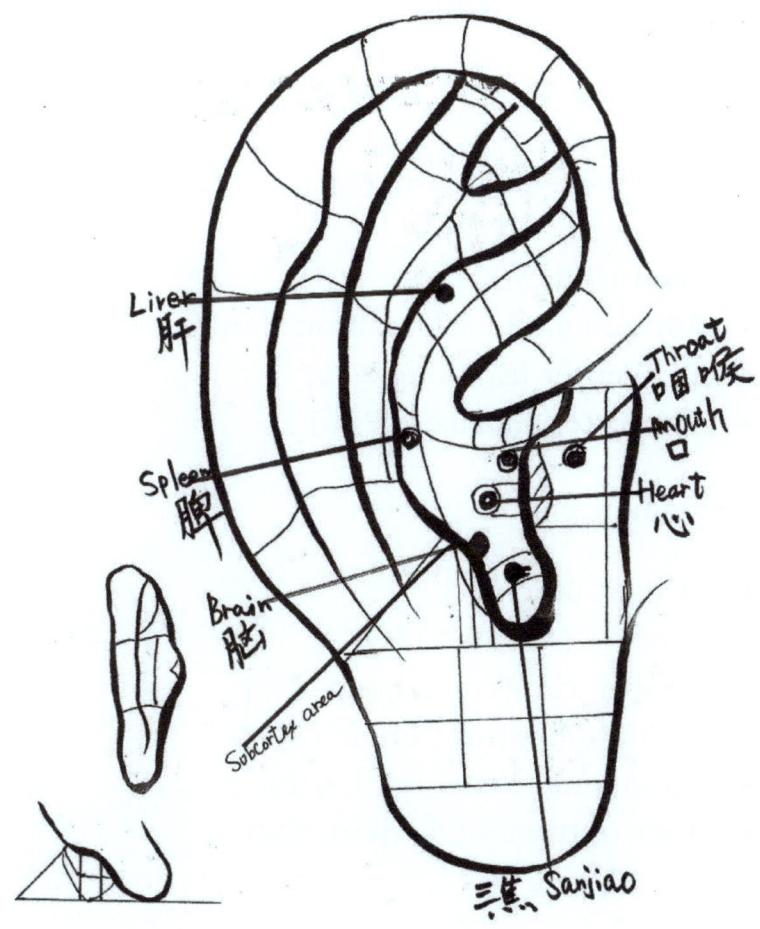

*Throat (Yanhou 咽喉)…covered

Section 4 Urogenital System Diseases

(1) Enuresis (Yiniao 遗尿)

Main points

- Bladder (Pangguang 膀胱)
- Kidney (Shen 肾)
- Liver (Gan 肝)
- Adrenal gland (Shenshangxian 肾上腺)
- Ear center (Erzhong 耳中)
- Subcortex (Pizhixia 皮质下)

Secondary points

- Occipit (Zhen 枕)
- Urethra (Niaodao 尿道)
- Central rim (Yuanzhong 缘中)
- Excitation point (Xingfen 兴奋)
- Endocrine (Neifenmi 内分泌)
- Apex of tragus (Pingjian 屏尖)

(1) Enuresis (Yiniao 遗尿)

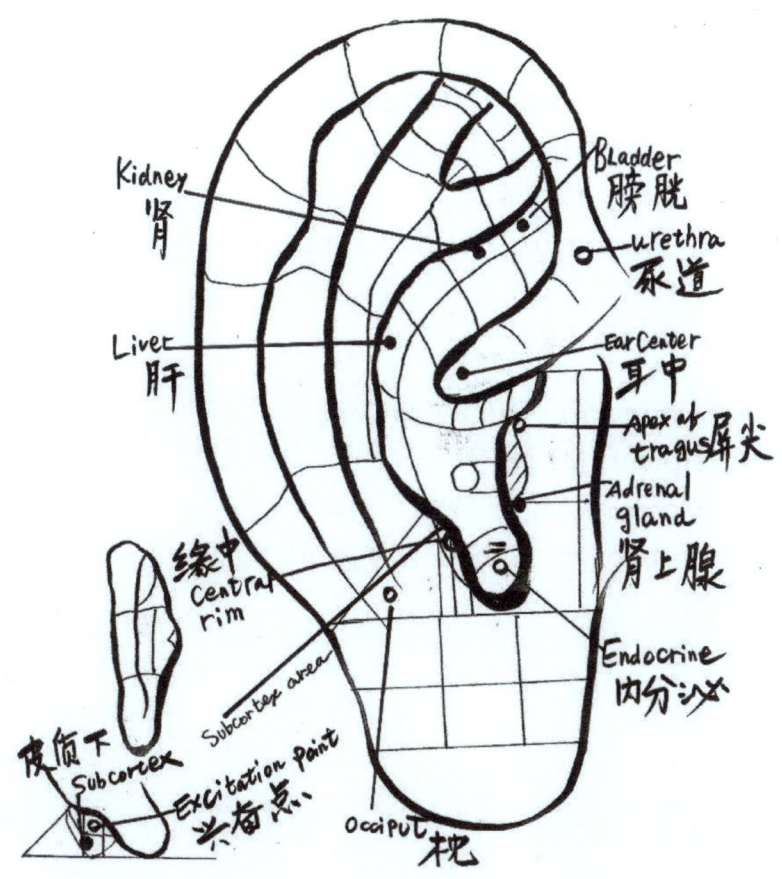

*Subcortex (Pizhixia 皮质下)··· covered

(2) Frequent Urination (Niaopin 尿频)

Main points

- Bladder (Pangguang 膀胱)
- Urethra (Niaodao 尿道)
- Kidney (Shen 肾)
- Central rim (Yuanzhong 缘中)

Secondary points

- Endocrine (Neifenmi 内分泌)
- Spleen (Pi 脾)
- Occipit (Zhen 枕)
- Subcortex (Pizhixia 皮质下)

(2) Frequent Urination (Niaopin 尿频)

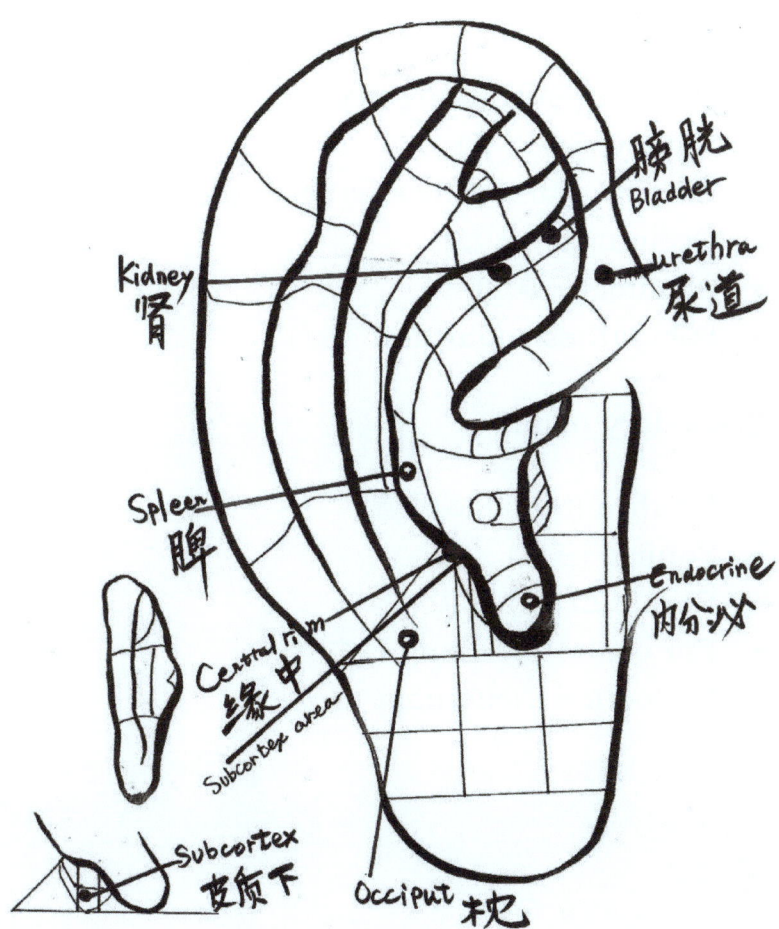

*Subcortex (Pizhixia 皮质下)⋯ covered

(3) Cystitis (Pangguangyan 膀胱炎)

Main points

- Bladder (Pangguang 膀胱)
- Kidney (Shen 肾)
- Adrenal gland (Shenshangxian 肾上腺)
- Occiput (Zhen 枕)
- Shenmen (神门)
- Sympathesis (Jiaogan 交感)

Secondary points

- Urethra (Niaodao 尿道)
- Sanjiao (三焦)
- Erjing (Erjian 耳尖)
- Ear center (Erzhong 耳中)
- Endocrine (Neifenmi 内分泌)

(3)Cystitis (Pangguangyan 膀胱炎)

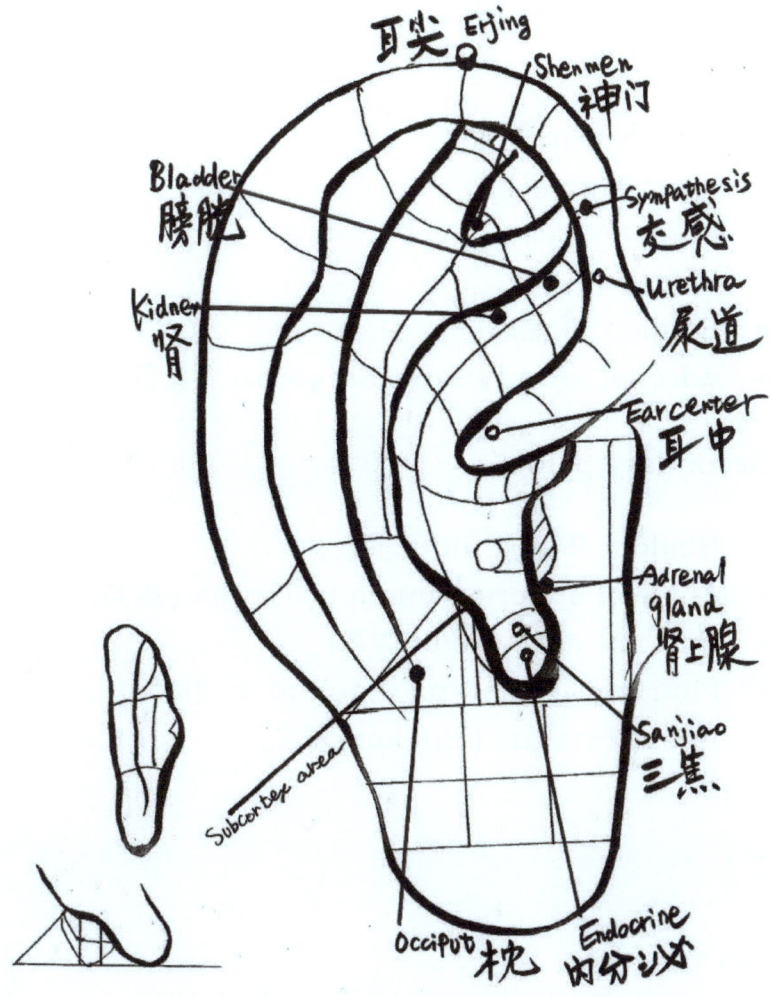

*Sympathesis (Jiaogan 交感)… covered

(4) Edema (Fuzhong 浮肿)

Main points

- Kidney (Shen 肾)
- Liver (Gan 肝)
- Lung (Fei 肺)
- Spleen (Pi 脾)
- Sanjiao (三焦)
- Adrenal grand (Shenshangxian 肾上腺)

Secondary points

- Bladder (Pangguang 膀胱)
- Angle of superior concha (Tingjiao 艇角)
- Internal nose (Neibi 内鼻)
- Pharynx and larynx (Yanhou 咽喉)
- Apex of tragus (Pingjian 屏尖)

(4) Edema (Fuzhong 浮肿)

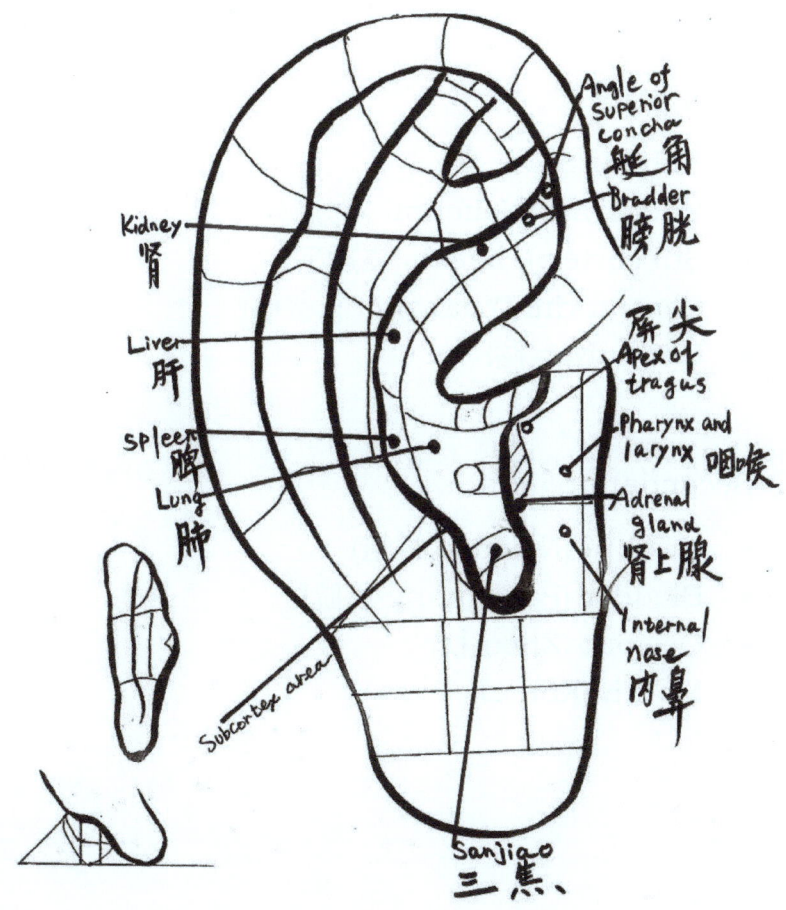

*Pharynx and larynx (Yanhou 咽喉)··· covered
* Internal nose (Neibi 内鼻)...covered

(5) Diabetes Insipidus (Niaobengzheng 尿崩症)

Main points

- Kidney (Shen 肾)
- Endocrine (Neifenmi 内分泌)
- Subcortex (Pizhixia 皮质下)
- Central rim (Yuanzhong 缘中)
- Brain (Nao 脑)

Secondary points

- Urethra (Niaodao 尿道)
- Bladder (Pangguang 膀胱)
- Occiput (Zhen 枕)
- Mouth (Kou 口)

(5) Diabetes Insipidus (Niaobengzheng 尿崩症)

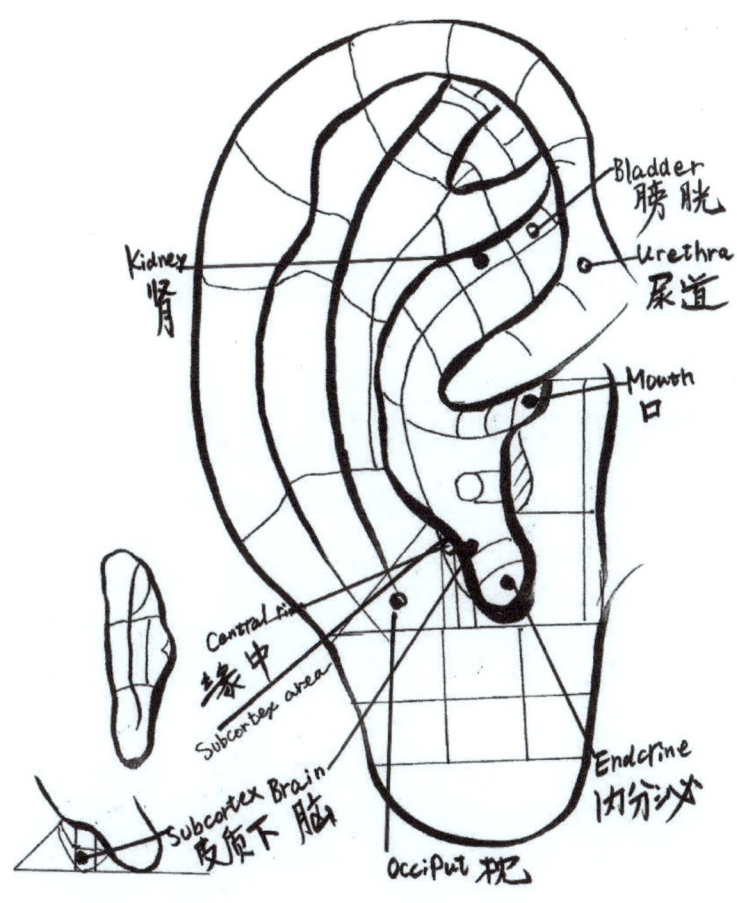

*Subcortex (Pizhixia 皮质下)··· covered

(6) Male Infertility (Nanxingburen 男性不妊)

Main points

- Internal genitals (Neishengzhiqi 内生殖器)
- Kidney (Shen 肾)
- Endocrine (Neifenmi 内分泌)
- Excitation point (Xingfendian 兴奋点)

Secondary points

- External genitals (Waishengzhiqi 外生殖器)
- Abdomen (Fu 腹)
- Testis (Gaowan 睾丸)

(6) Male Infertility (Nanxingburen 男性不妊)

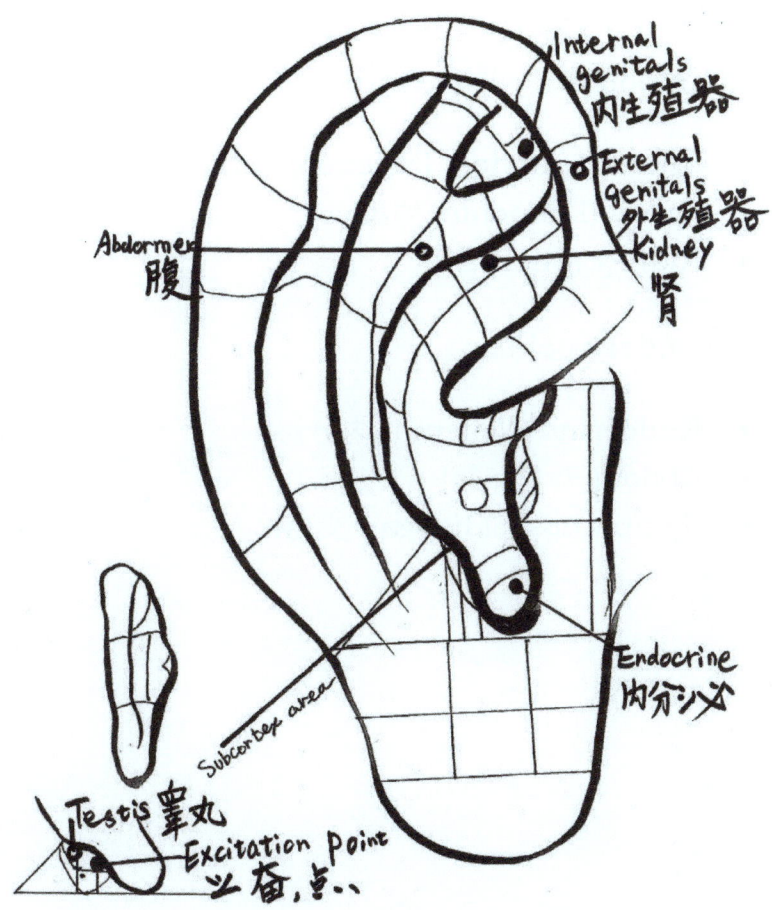

* Testis (Gaowan 睾丸)… Covered
* Excitation point (Xingfendian 兴奋点)… covered

(7) Female Infertility (Nüxingburen 女性不妊)

Main points

- Internal genitals (Neishengzhiqi 内生殖器)
- Ovary (Luanchao 卵巢)
- Kidney (Shen 肾)

Secondary points

- Endocrine (Neifenmi 内分泌)
- Abdomen (Fu 腹)
- Sympathesis (Jiaogan 交感)

(7) Female Infertility (Nüxingburen 女性不妊)

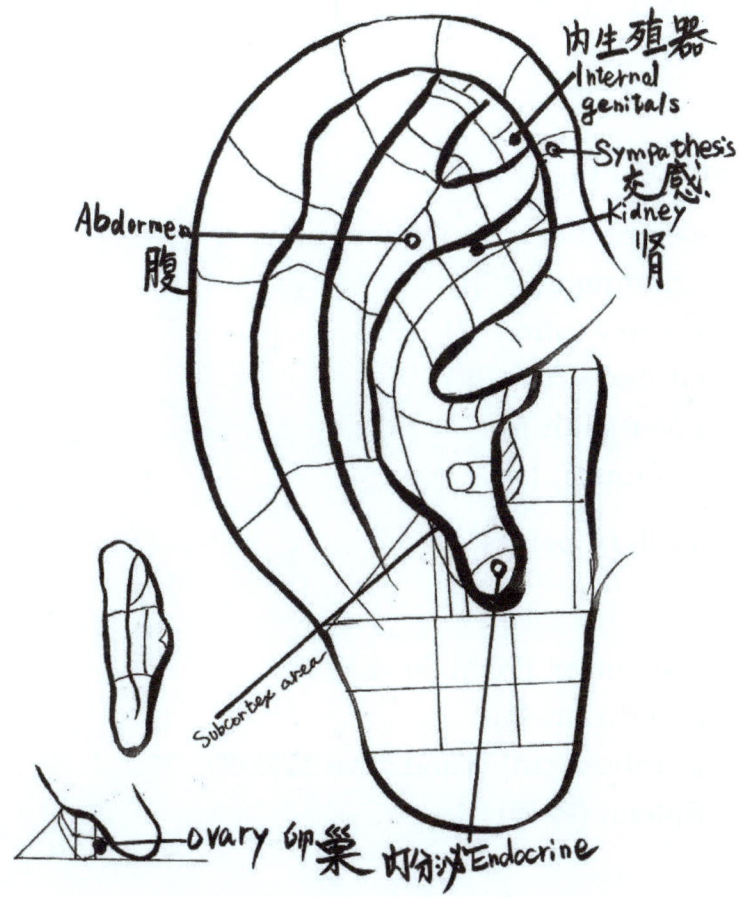

内生殖器
Internal
genitals

Sympathesis
交感.

Kidney
肾

Abdormen
腹

Subcortex area

Ovary 卵巣　内分沙 Endocrine

*Sympathesis (Jiaogan 交感)... covered
*Ovary (Luanchao 卵巣)... covered

CHAPTER 2. Surgical Diseases

(1) Sciatica (Zuogushenjingtong 坐骨神经痛)

Main points

- Sciatic nerve (Zuogushenjing 坐骨神经)
- Shenmen (神门)
- Kidney (Shen 肾)
- Gluteus (Tun 臀)
- Liver (Gan 肝)
- Occiput (Zhen 枕)

Secondary points

- Subcortex (Pizhixia 皮质下)
- Hip (Kuan 髋)
- Lumbosacral (Yaodizhui 腰骶椎)
- Spleen (Pi 脾)

(1) Sciatica (Zuogushenjingtong 坐骨神经痛)

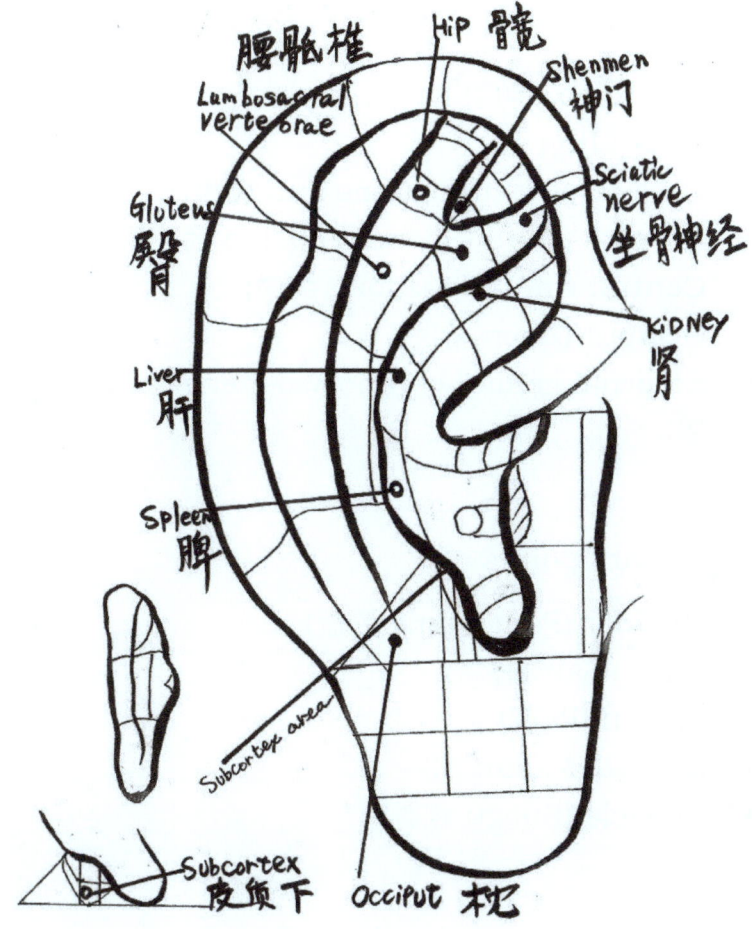

*Subcortex (Pizhixia 皮质下) ⋯ covered

(2) Stiffness of the Neck (Laozhen 落枕)

Main points

- Shenmen (神门)
- Neck (Jing 颈)
- Cervical vertebrae (Jingzhui 颈椎)
- Adrenal gland (Shenshangxian 肾上腺)
- Central rim (Yuanzhong 缘中)
- Occiput (Zhen 枕)
- External genital organ (Waishengzhiqi 外生殖器)

Secondary points

- Bladder (Pangguang 膀胱)
- Liver (Gan 肝)
- Spleen (Pi 脾)
- Shoulder (Jian 肩)
- Clavicle (Suogu 锁骨)

(2) Stiffness of the Neck (Laozhen 落枕)

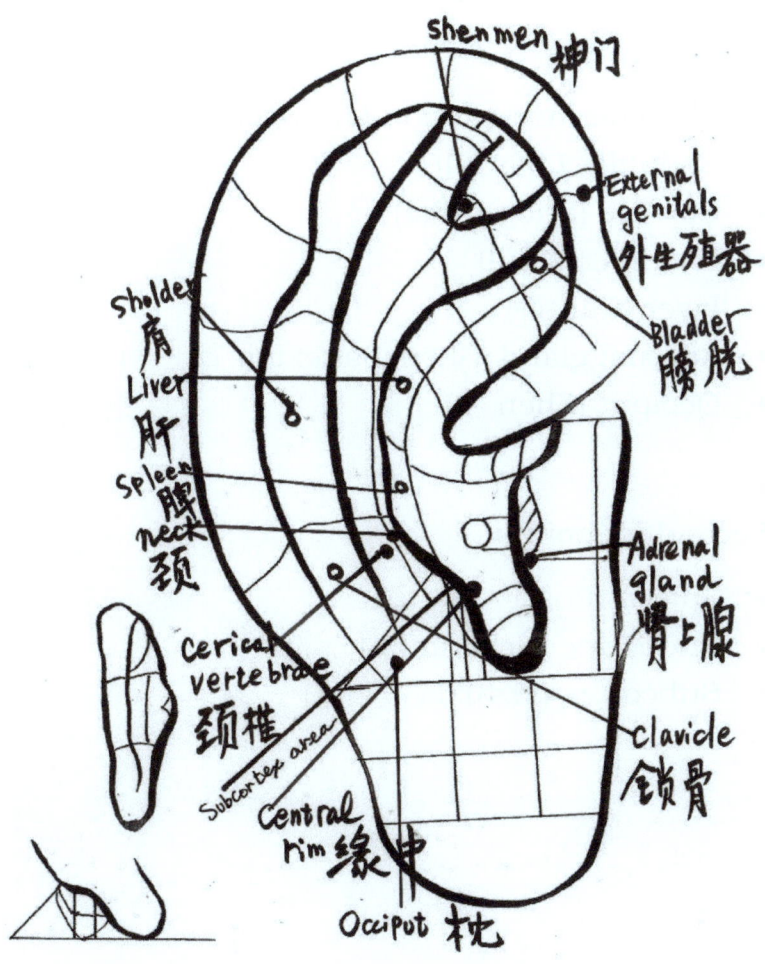

(3) Periarthritis of Shoulder (Jianguanjiezhouweiyan 肩关节周围炎)

Main points

- Shoulder articulation (Jianguanjie 肩关节)
- Shoulder (Jian 肩)
- Clavicle (Suogu 锁骨)
- Shenmen (神门)
- Liver (Gan 肝)
- Adrenal gland (Shenshangxian 肾上腺)
- Occiput (Zhen 枕)

Secondary points

- Spleen (Pi 脾)
- Endocrine (Neifenmi 内分泌)
- Subcortex (Pizhixia 皮质下)

(3) Periarthritis of Shoulder
(Jianguanjiezhouweiyan 肩关节周围炎)

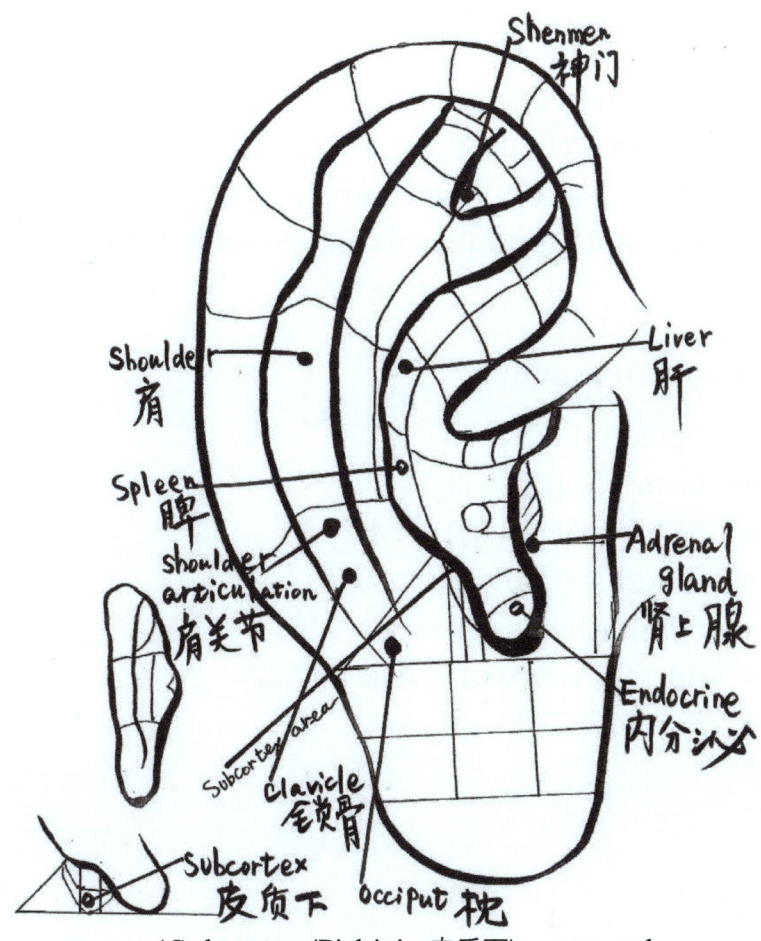

*Subcortex (Pizhixia 皮质下) … covered

(4) Acute Lumbar Sprain (Jixingcuoshang 急性挫伤)

Main points

- Shenmen (神门)
- Gluteus (Tun 臀)
- Lumbosacral vertebrae (Yaodizhui 腰骶椎))
- Adrenal gland (Shenshangxian 肾上腺)

Secondary points

- Spleen (Pi 脾)
- Liver (Gan 肝)
- Kidney (Shen 肾)
- Bladder (Pangguang 膀胱)
- Sympathesis (Jiaogan 交感)
- Apex of tragus (Pingjian 屏尖)
- Sanjiao (三焦)

(4) Acute Lumbar Sprain (Jixingcuoshang 急性挫伤)

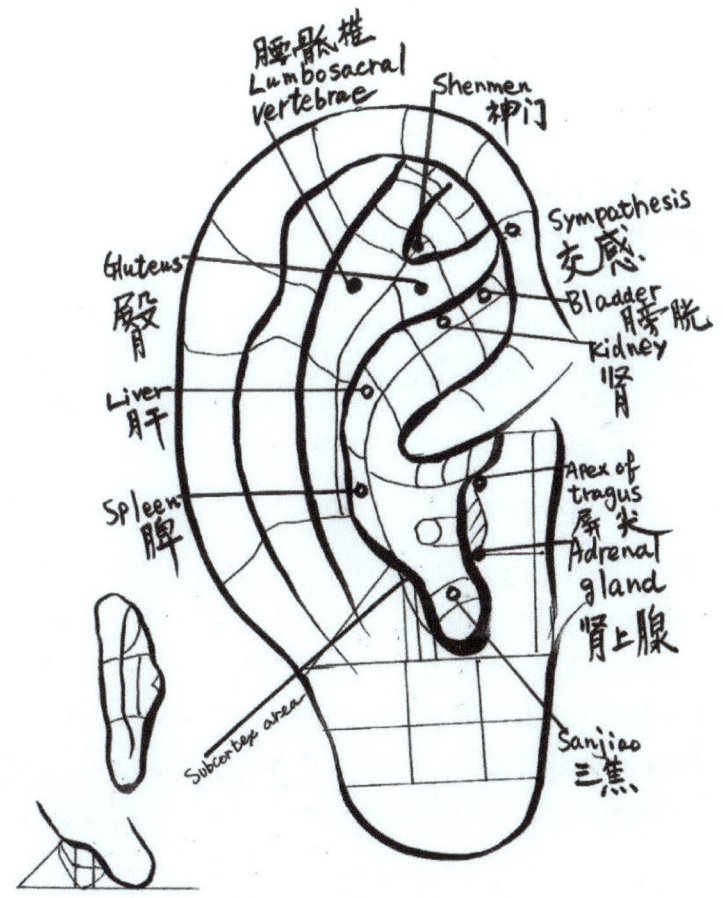

*Sympathesis (Jiaogan 交感) … covered

(5) Cervical Spondylosis (Jingzhuibing 颈椎病)

Main points

- Shenmen (神门)
- Neck (Jingzhui 颈椎)
- Kidney (Shen 肾)
- Sympathesis (Jiaogan 交感)
- Liver (Gan 肝)
- Cervical Vertebrae (Jing 颈)
- Subcortex (Pizhixia 皮质下)

Secondary points

- Shoulder (Jian 肩)
- Occiput (zhen 枕)
- Central rim (Yuanzhong 缘中)
- Endocrine (Neifenmi 内分泌)
- Forehead (E 额)
- External ear (Waier 外耳)

(5) Cervical Spondylosis (Jingzhuibing 颈椎病)

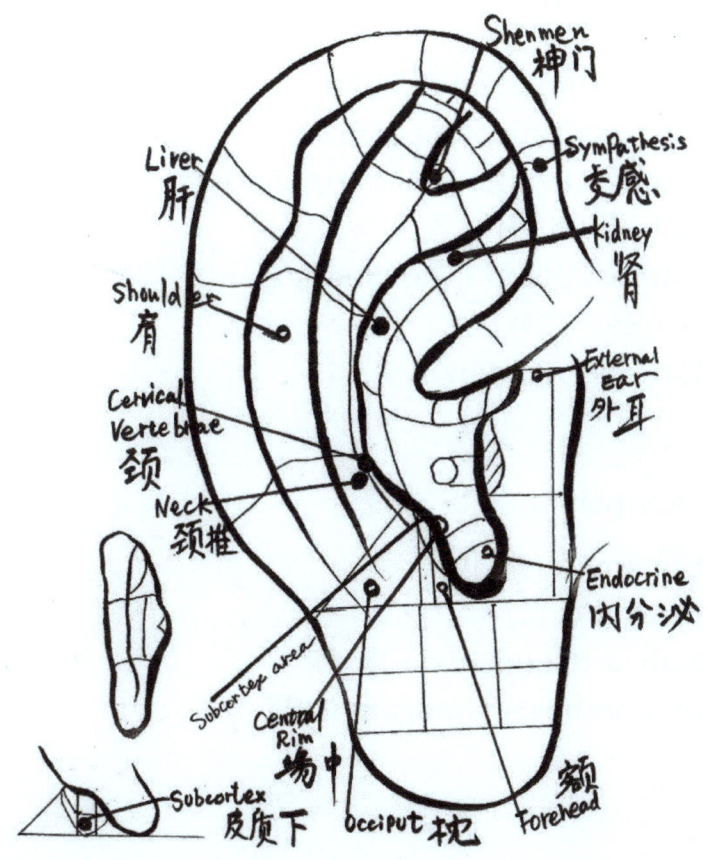

*Sympathesis (Jiaogan 交感) … covered
*Subcortex (Pizhixia 皮质下) … covered

(6) (Hemorrhoid (Zhichuang 痔疮)

Main points

- Anus (Gangmen 肛门)
- Rectum (Zhichang 直肠)
- Large Intestine (Dachang 大肠)
- Spleen (Pi 脾)
- Adrenal gland (Shenshangxian 肾上腺)
- Sanjiao (三焦)
- Ear apex (Erjian 耳尖)

Secondary points

- Shenmen (神门)
- Lung (Fei 肺)
- Subcortex (Pizhixia 皮质下)
- Sympathesis (Jiaogan 交感)

(6) (Hemorrhoid (Zhichuang 痔疮)

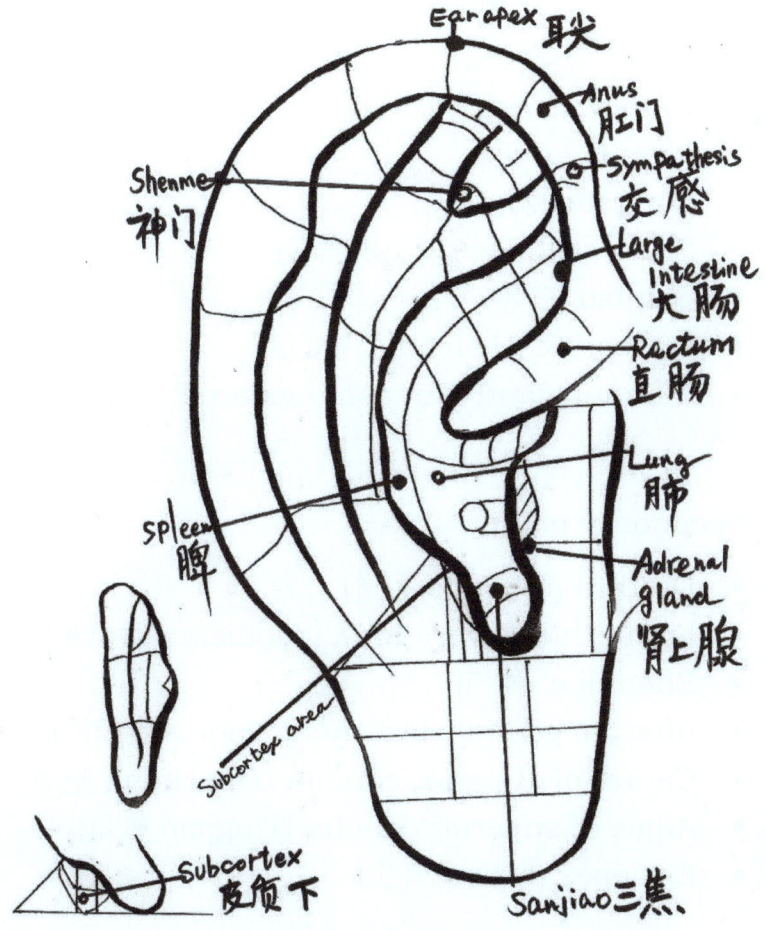

*Sympathesis (Jiaogan 交感) … covered
*Subcortex (Pizhixia 皮质下) … covered

(7) Bi Syndromes (Bi Zhenghou Bi 证候)

Main points

- Kidney (Shen 肾)
- Liver (Gan 肝)
- Lung (Fei 肺)
- Subcortex (Pizhixia 皮质下)
- Sanjiao (三焦)
- Endocrine (Neifenmi 内分泌)
- Adrenal gland (Shenshangxian 肾上腺)

Secondary points

- Urethra (Niaodao 尿道)
- Lumbosacral vertebrae (Yaodizhui 腰骶椎)
- Shenmen (神门)
- Internal genitals (Neishengzhiqi 内生殖器)
- Center of superior concha (Tingzhong 艇中)
- Angle of superior concha (Tingjiao 艇角)
- Ear apex (Erjian 耳尖)

(7) Bi Syndromes (Bi Zhenghou Bi 证候)

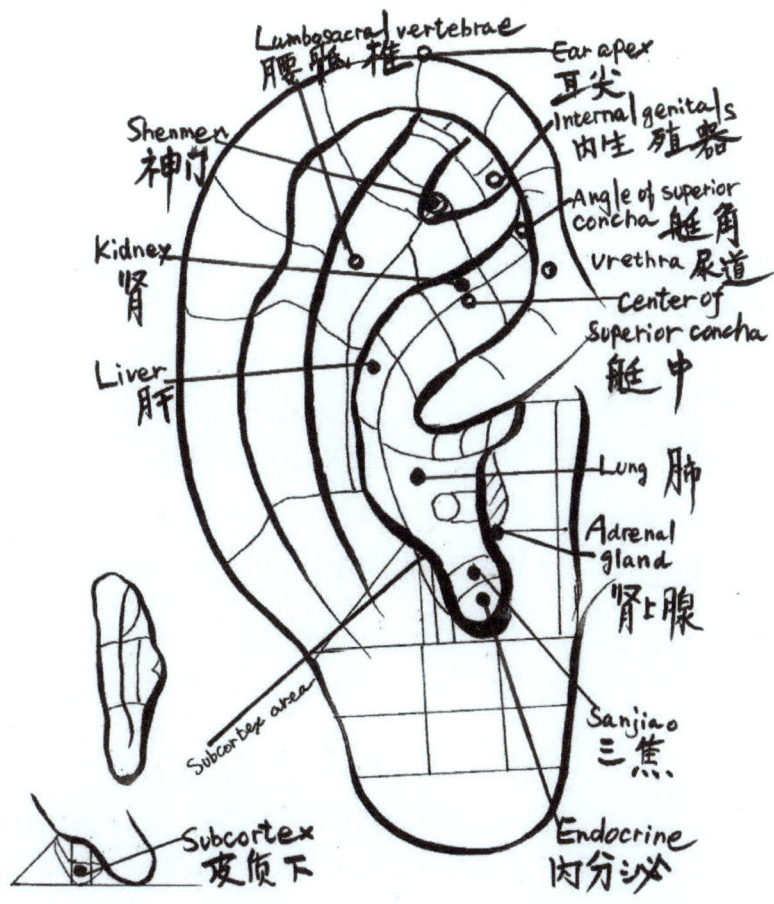

*Subcortex (Pizhixia 皮质下) … covered

(8) Heel pain (Zugentong 足跟痛)

Main points

- Heel (Gen 跟)
- Kidney (Shen 肾)
- Subcortex (Pizhixia 皮质下)

Secondary points

- Shenmen (神门)
- Bladder (Pangguang 膀胱)

(8) Heel pain (Zugentong 足跟痛)

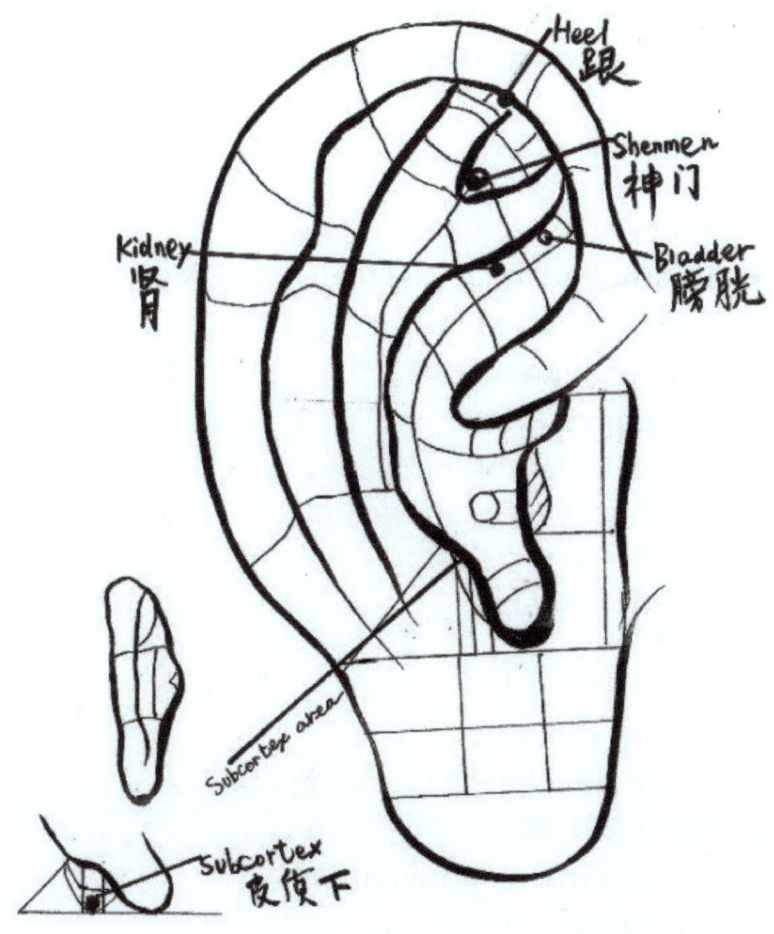

*Subcortex (Pizhixia 皮质下) …covered

CHAPTER 3. Gynecology Diseases

(1) Menopausal Syndrome (Gengnianqizonghezheng 更年期综合症)

Main points

- Endocrine (Neifenmi 内分泌)
- Internal genitals (Neishengzhiqi 内生殖器)
- Sympathesis (Jiaogan 交感)
- Ovary (Luanchao 卵巢)
- Shenmen (神门)
- Adrenal gland (Shenshangxian 肾上腺)
- Subcortex (Pizhixia 皮质下)

Secondary points

- Heart (Xin 心)
- Kidney (Shen 肾)
- Small Intestine (Xiaochang 小肠)
- Lung (Fei 肺)
- Apex of tragus (Pingjian 屏尖)
- Liver (Gan 肝)

(1) Menopausal Syndrome
(Gengnianqizonghezheng 更年期综合症)

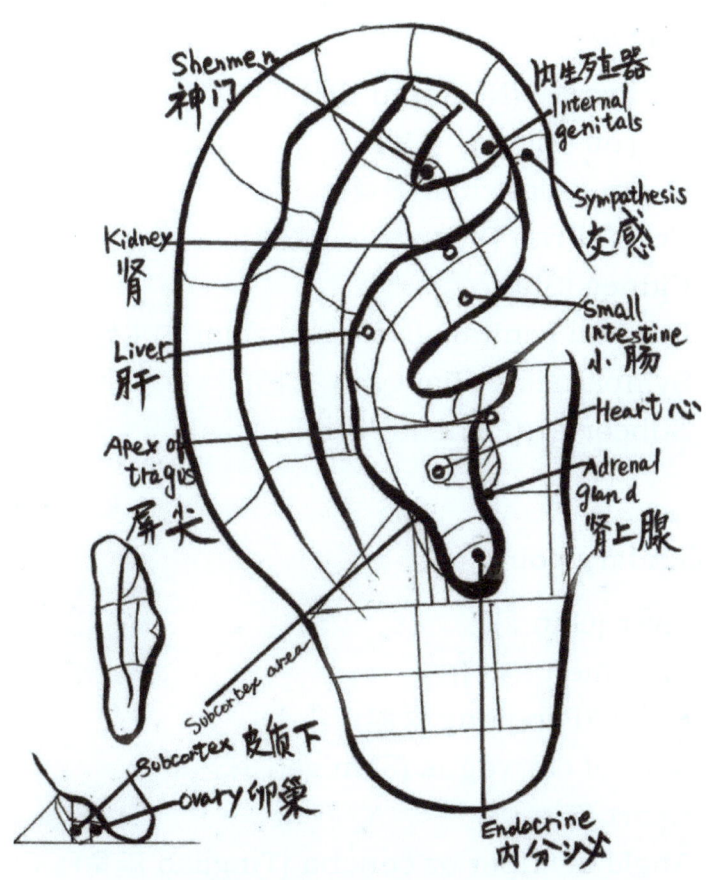

*Sympathesis (Jiaogan 交感) ... covered
*Subcortex (Pizhixia 皮质下) ... covered
*Ovary (Luanchao 卵巢) ... covered

(2) Dysmenorrhea (Tongjing 痛经)

Main points

- Endocrine (Neifenmi 内分泌)
- Uterus (Zigong 子宫)
- Ovary (Luanchao 卵巢)
- Central rim (Yuanzhong 缘中)
- Kidney (Shen 肾)
- Internal genitals (Neishengzhiqi 内生殖器)
- Sympathesis (Jiaoggan 交感)
- Subcortex (Pizhixia 皮质下)

Secondary points

- Liver (Gan 肝)
- Shenmen (神门)
- Pelvis (Penqiang 盆腔)
- Root of ear vagus (Ermigen 耳迷根)
- Heart (Xin 心)
- Angle of superior concha (Tingjiao 艇角)

(2) Dysmenorrhea (Tongjing 痛经)

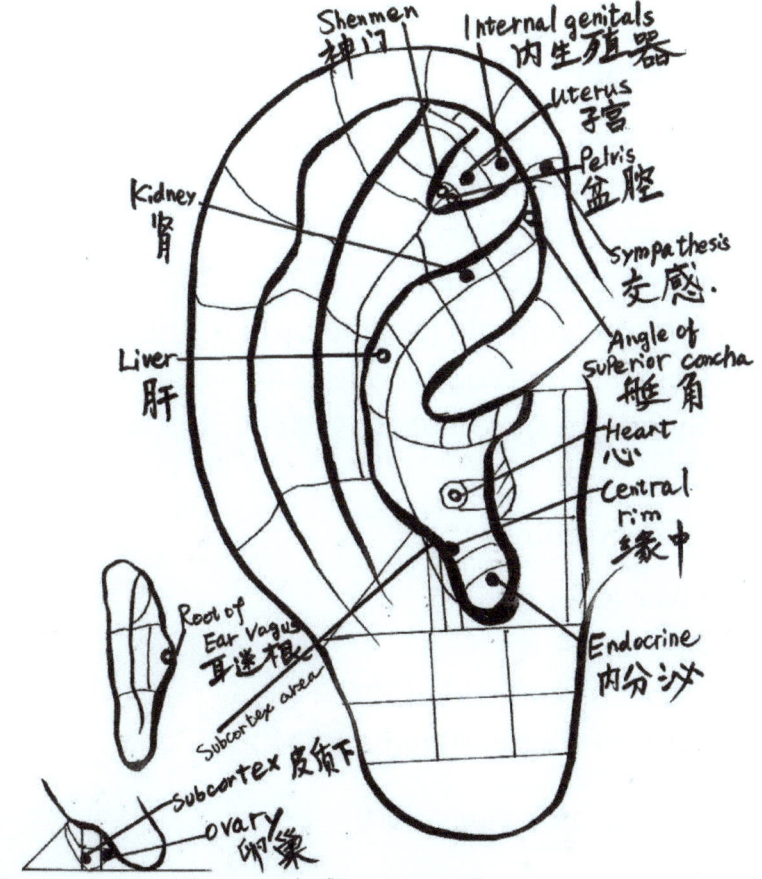

*Sympathesis (Jiaogan 交感) ⋯ covered
*Subcortex (Pizhixia 皮质下) ⋯ covered
*Ovary (Luanchao 卵巢) ⋯ covered
*Root of Ear vagus (Ermigen 耳迷根) ...ear behind

(3) Irregular Menstruation (Yuejingbutiao 月经不调)

Main points

- Endocrine (Neifenmi 内分泌)
- Kidney (Shen 肾)
- Ovary (Luanchao 卵巢)
- Pelvis (Pengu 盆骨)
- Internal genitals (Neishengzhiqi 内生殖器)
- Central rim (Yuanzhong 缘中)
- Sympathesis (Jiaogan 交感)

Secondary points

- Liver (Gan 肝)
- Spleen (Pi 脾)
- Subcortex (Pizhixia 皮质下)
- Apex of tragus (Pingjian 屏尖)

(3) Irregular Menstruation (Yuejingbutiao 月经不调)

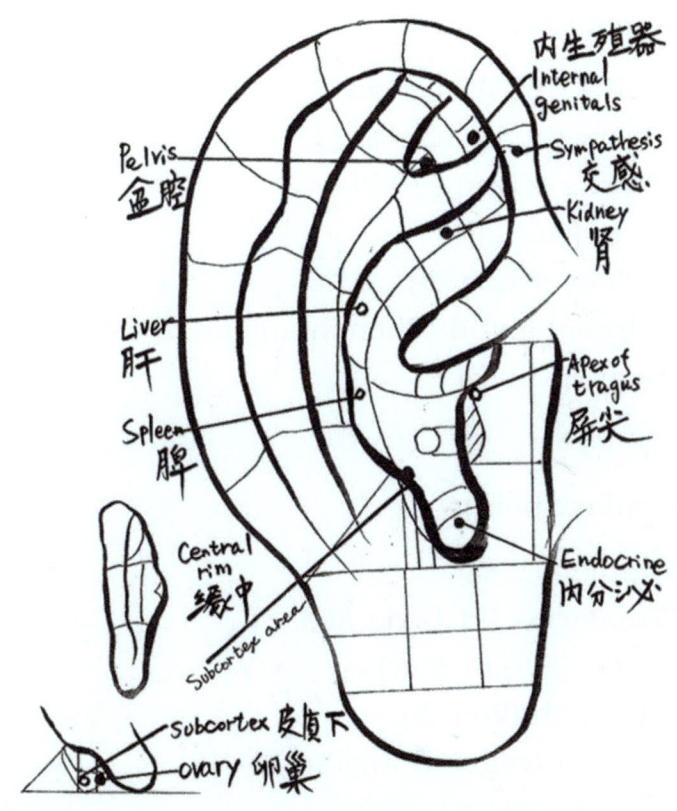

*Sympathesis (Jiaogan 交感)... covered
*Subcortex (Pizhixia 皮质下)... covered
*Ovary (Luanchao 卵巢)... covered

(4) Amenorrhea (Bijing 闭经)

Main points

- Endocrine (Neifenmi 内分泌)
- Ovary (Luanchao 卵巢)
- Uterus (Zigong 子宫)
- Liver (Gan 肝)
- Kidney (Shen 肾)
- Adrenal gland (Shenshianxian 肾上腺)
- Heart (Xin 心)

Secondary points

- Sanjiao (三焦)
- Subcortex (Pizhixia 皮质下)
- Pelvis (Pengu 盆骨)
- Stomach (Wei 胃)
- Apex of tragus (Pingjian 屏尖)

4) Amenorrhea (Bijing 闭经)

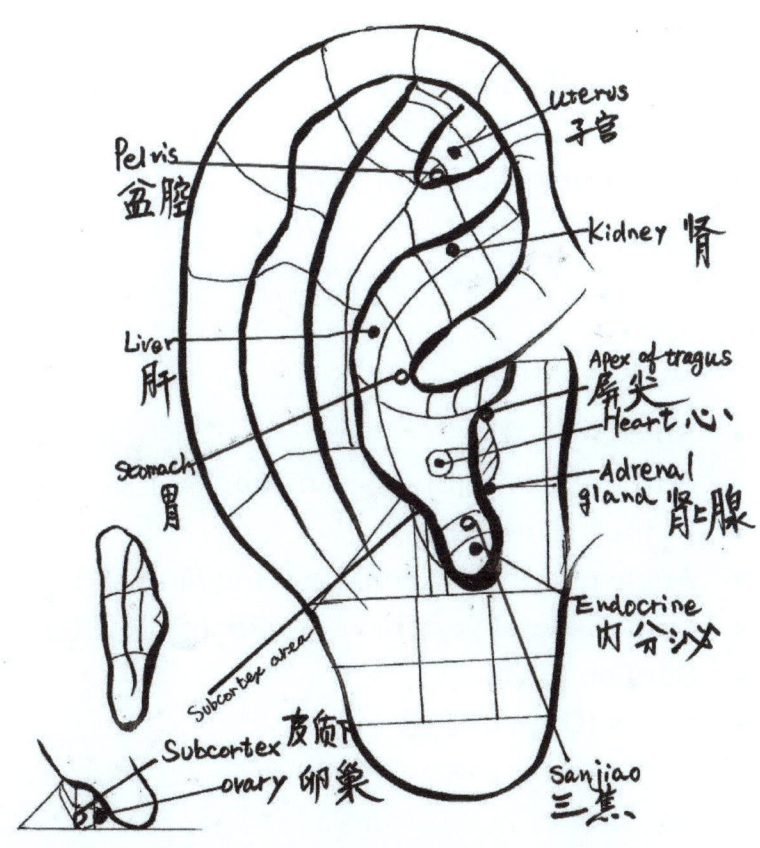

Pelvis 盆腔
Uterus 子宫
Kidney 肾
Liver 肝
Apex of tragus 屏尖
Heart 心
Adrenal gland 肾上腺
Stomach 胃
Endocrine 内分泌
Subcortex area
Subcortex 皮质下
ovary 卵巢
Sanjiao 三焦

*Subcortex (Pizhixia 皮质下) … covered
*Ovary (Luanchao 卵巢) … covered

(5) Leukorrhea (Baidaizengduo 白带增多)

Main points

- Uterus (Zigong 子宫)
- Ovary (Luanchao 卵巢)
- Endocrine (Neifenmi 内分泌)

Secondary points

- Spleen (Pi 脾)
- Adrenal gland (Shenshangxian 肾上腺)
- Kidney (Shen 肾)
- Angle of superior concha (Tingjiao 艇角)
- Lumbosacral vertebrae (Yaodizhui 腰骶椎)
- Sanjiao (三焦)
- Pelvis (Gupen 骨盆)

(5) Leukorrhea (Baidaizengduo 白带增多)

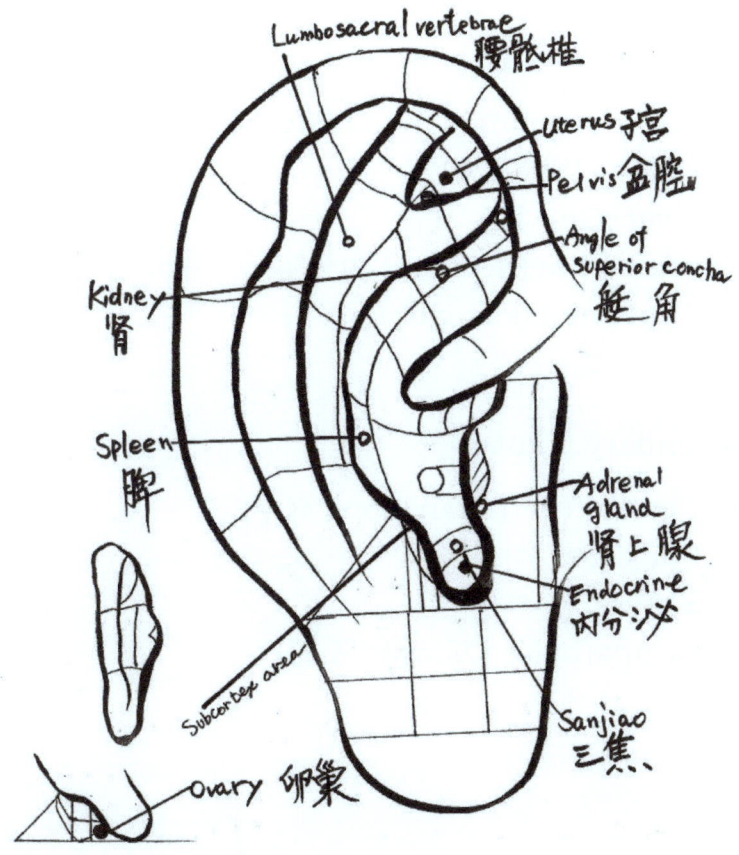

Lumbosacral vertebrae 腰骶椎
Uterus 子宫
Pelvis 盆腔
Angle of superior concha 艇角
Kidney 肾
Spleen 脾
Adrenal gland 肾上腺
Endocrine 内分泌
Subcortex area
Sanjiao 三焦
Ovary 卵巢

*Ovary (Luanchao 卵巢) ... covered

(6) Hysteroptosis (Zigongdiaowang 子宫凋亡)

Main points

- Internal genitals (Neishengzhiqi 内生殖器)
- Kidney (Shen 肾)
- Liver (Gan 肝)
- Endocrine (Neifenmi 内分泌)
- Subcortex (Pizhixia 皮质下)

Secondary points

- Central rim (Yuanzhong 缘中)
- Lung (Fei 肺)
- Sanjiao (三焦)
- Sympathesis (Jiaogan 交感)

(6) Hysteroptosis (Zigongdiaowang 子宫凋亡)

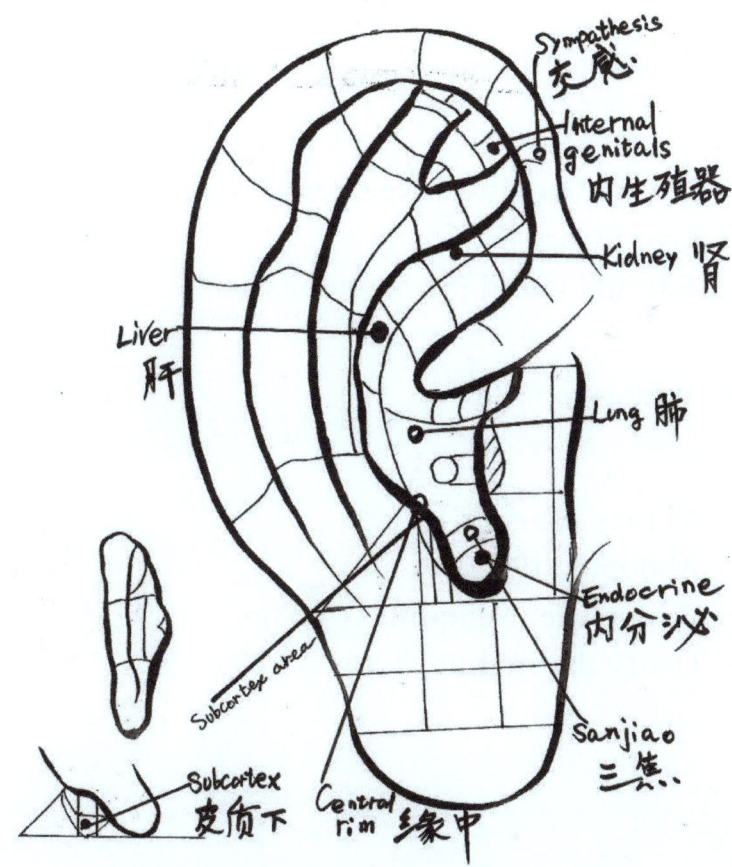

'Sympathesis (Jiaogan 交感)··· covered
*Subcortex (Pizhixia 皮质下)··· covered

(7) Menorrhagia (Yuejingguoduo 月经过多)

Main points

- Internal genitals (Neishengzhiqi 内生殖器)
- Liver (Gan 肝)
- Adrenal gland (Shenshangxian 肾上腺)

Secondary points

- Kidney (Shen 肾)
- Abdomen (Fu 腹)
- Endocrine (Neifenmi 内分泌)
- Ovary (Luanchao 卵巢)

(7) Menorrhagia (Yuejingguoduo 月经过多)

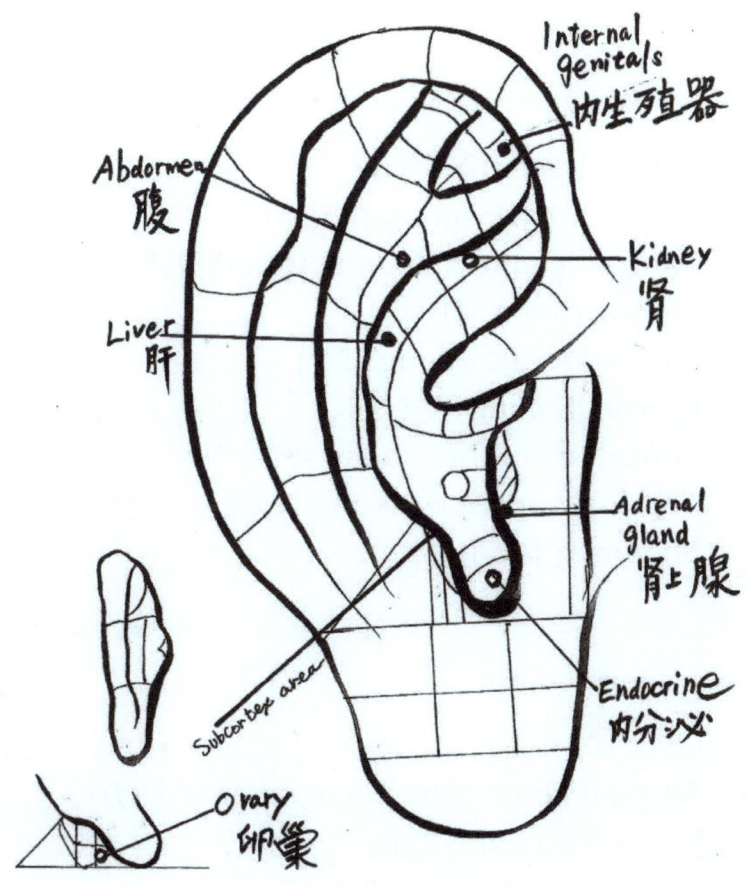

*Ovary (Luanchao 卵巢) ... covered

(8) Functional Uterine Bleeding (Gongneng xing zigong chuxie 功能性子宫出血)

Main points

- Ovary (Luanchao 卵巢)
- Endocrine (Neifenmi 内分泌)
- Internal genitals (Neishengzhiqi 内生殖器)
- Kidney (Shen 肾)
- Ear Center (Erzhong 耳中)
- Uterus (Zigong 子宫)
- Central rim (Yuanzhong 缘中)
- Angle of superior concha (Tingjiao 艇角)
- Shenmen (神门)

Secondary points

- Liver (Gan 肝)
- Adrenal gland (Shenshangxian 肾上腺)
- Pelvis (Penqiang 盆腔)
- Subcortex (Pizhixia 皮质下)
- Lung (Fei 肺)

(8) Functional Uterine Bleeding (Gongneng xing zigong chuxie 功能性子宫出血)

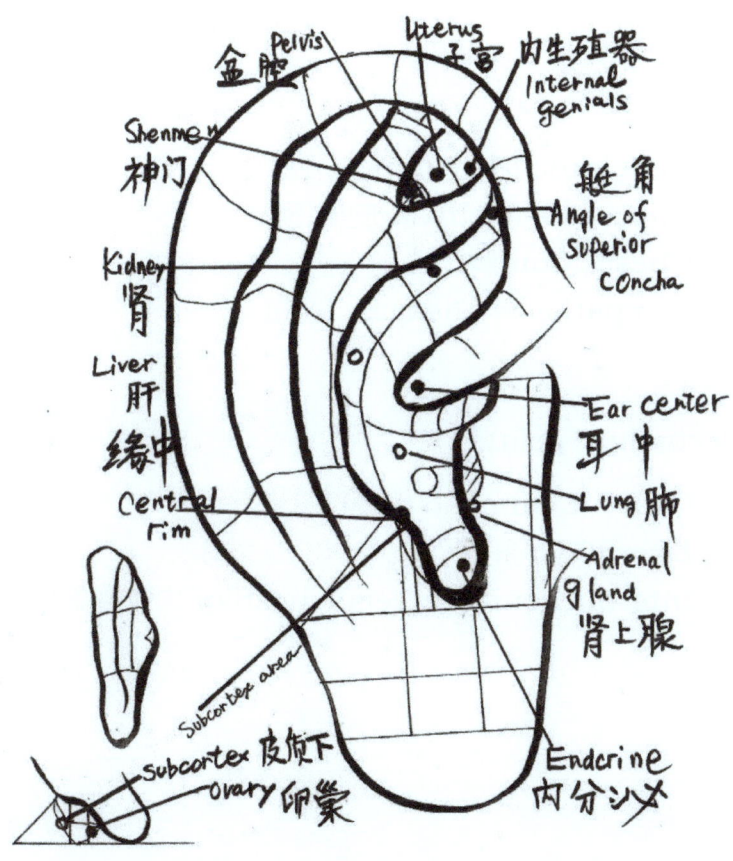

*Subcortex (Pizhixia 皮质下) ... covered
*Ovary (Luanchao 卵巢) ... covered

(9) Hyperplasia of Mammary Glands (Ruxian zengsheng 乳腺增生)

Main points

- Endocrine (Neifenmi 内分泌)
- Subcortex (Pizhixia 皮质下)
- Chest (Xion 胸)
- Sympathesis (Jiaogan 交感)

Secondary points

- Ovary (Luanchao 卵巢)
- Liver (Gan 肝)
- Internal genitals (Neishengzhiqi 内生殖器)

(9) Hyperplasia of Mammary Glands (Ruxian zengsheng 乳腺增生)

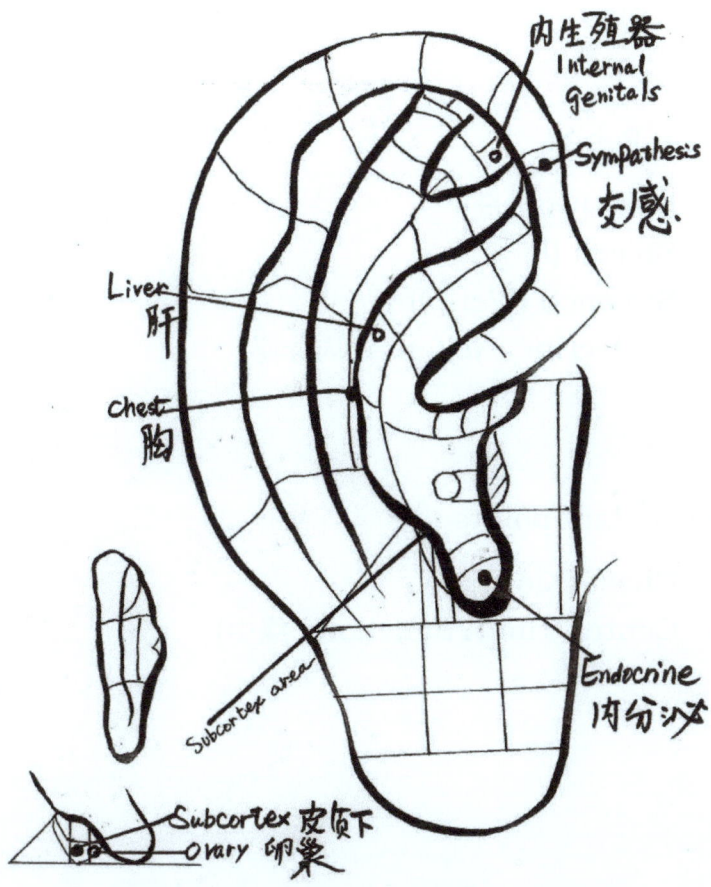

'Sympathesis (Jiaogan 交感) … covered
*Subcortex (Pizhixia 皮质下) … covered
*Ovary (Luanchao 卵巢) … covered

(10) Insufficient Lactation (Burubuzu 哺乳不足)

Main Points

- Liver (Gan 肝)
- Spleen (Pi 脾)
- Stomach (Wei 胃)
- Endocrine (Neifenmi 内分泌)

Secondary points

- Chest (Xion 胸)
- Central rim (Yuanzhong 缘中)

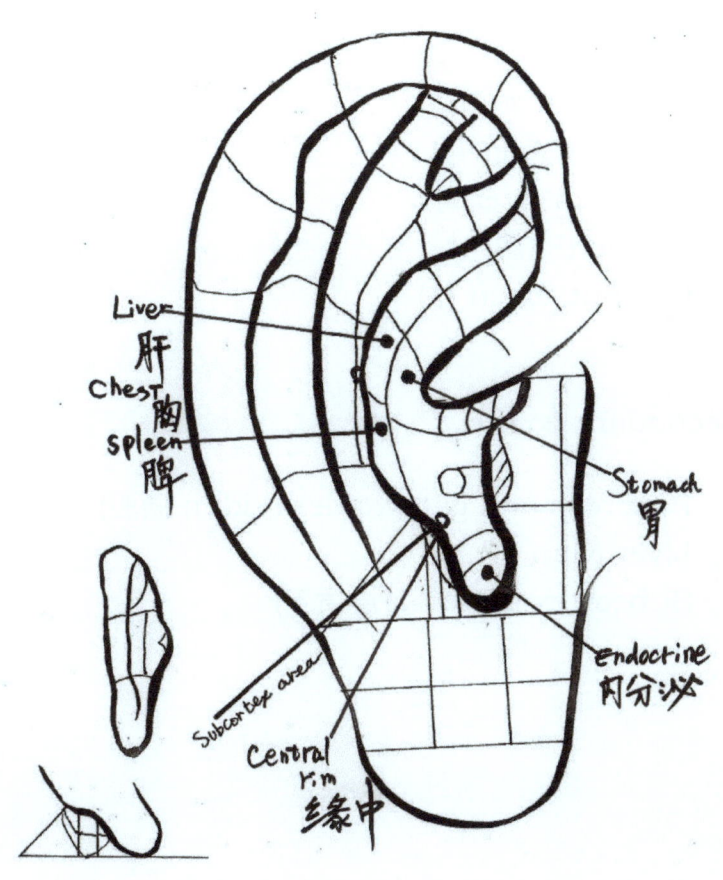

(10) Insufficient Lactation (Burubuzu 哺乳不足)

(11) Morning Sickness (Yuntu 孕吐)

Main points

- Shenmen (神门)
- Kidney (Shen 肾)
- Stomach (Wei 胃)
- Spleen (Pi 脾)
- Occiput (Zhen 枕)

Secondary points

- Pancreas and gallbladder (Yidan 胰胆)
- Liver (Gan 肝)
- Subcortex (Pizhixia 皮质下)

(11) Morning Sickness (Yuntu 孕吐)

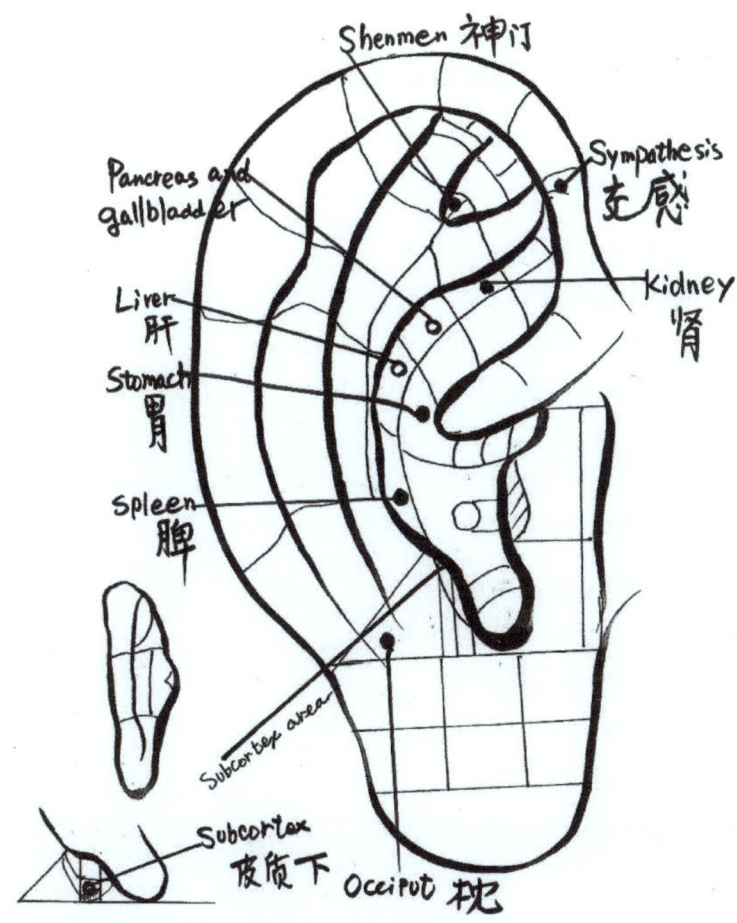

'Sympathesis (Jiaogan 交感)… covered
*Subcortex (Pizhixia 皮质下)… covered

CHAPTER 4. Eye, Ear, Nose and Throat Diseases

(1) Epistaxis (Bichuxie 鼻出血)

Main points

- Lung (Fei 肺)
- Forehead (E 额)
- Internal nose (Neibi 内鼻)
- Adrenal gland (Shenshangxian 肾上腺)

Secondary points

- Kidney (Shen 肾)
- Ear apex (Erjian 耳尖)
- Shenmen (神门)
- Central rim (Yuanzhong 缘中)
- Spleen (Pi 脾)
- External nose (Waibi 外鼻)

(1) Epistaxis (Bichuxie 鼻出血)

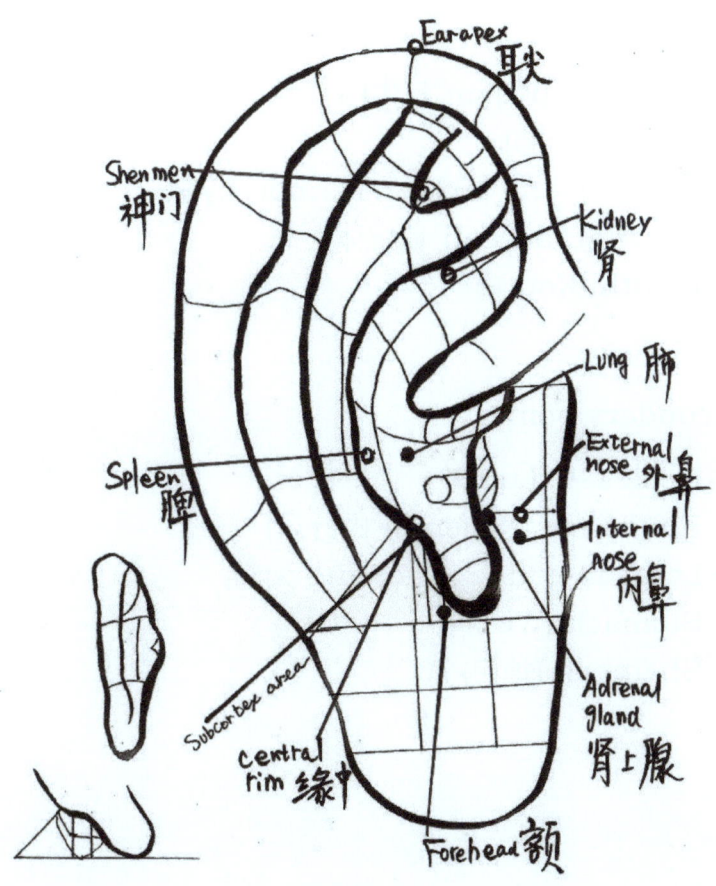

*Internal nose (Neibi 内鼻) … covered

(2) Tonsillitis (Biantaotiyan 扁桃体炎)

Main points

- Ear apex (Erjian 耳尖)
- Lung (Fei 肺)
- Pharynx and larynx (Yanhou 咽喉)
- Tonsil (Biantaoti 扁桃体)
- Mouth (Kou 口)

Secondary points

- Helix 1-4 (Lun 轮)
- Endocrine (Neifenmi 内分泌)
- Large intestine (Dachang 大肠)
- Stomach (Wei 胃)
- Shenmen (神门)

(2) Tonsillitis (Biantaotiyan 扁桃体炎)

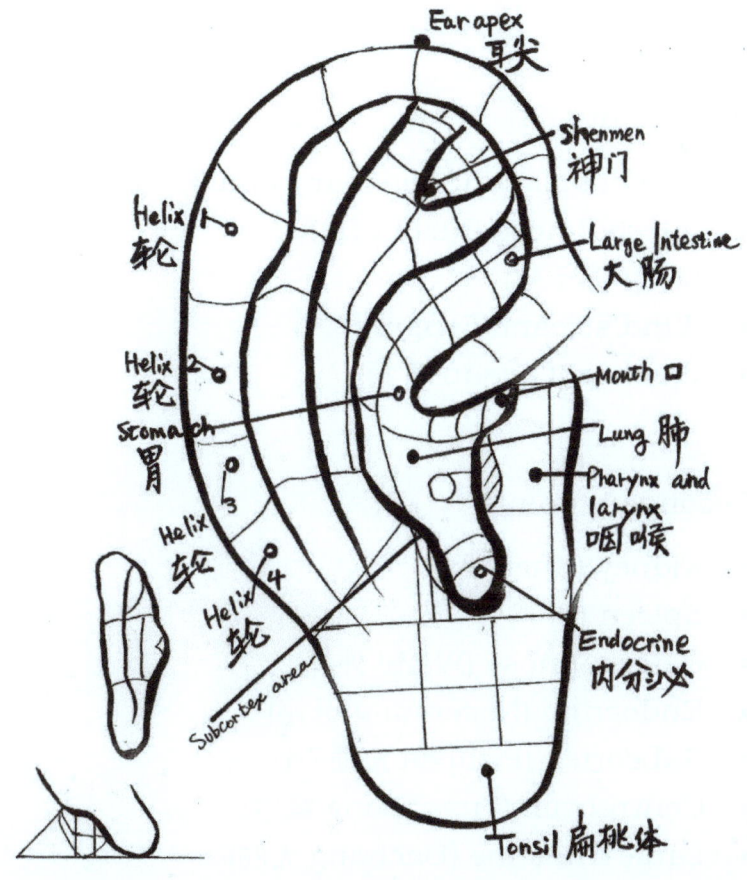

Ear apex 耳尖
Shenmen 神门
Large Intestine 大肠
Helix 轮 1
Helix 轮 2
Mouth 口
Stomach 胃
Lung 肺
Pharynx and larynx 咽喉
Helix 轮 3
Helix 轮 4
Subcortex area
Endocrine 内分泌
Tonsil 扁桃体

*Pharynx And larynx (Yanhou 咽喉) …covered

(3) Allergic Rhinitis (Guominxingbiyan 过敏性鼻炎)

Main points

- Adrenal gland (Shenshangxian 肾上腺)
- Internal nose (Neibi 内鼻)
- Lung (Fei 肺)
- Wind stream (Fengxi 风溪)
- Trachea (Qiguan 气管)

Secondary points

- Kidney (Shen 肾)
- Spleen (Pi 脾)
- External nose (Waibi 外鼻)
- Endocrine (Neifenmi 内分泌)
- Subcortex (Pizhixia 皮质下)
- Central rim (Yuanzhong 缘中)
- Large intestine (Dachang 大肠)

(3) Allergic Rhinitis (Guominxingbiyan 过敏性鼻炎)

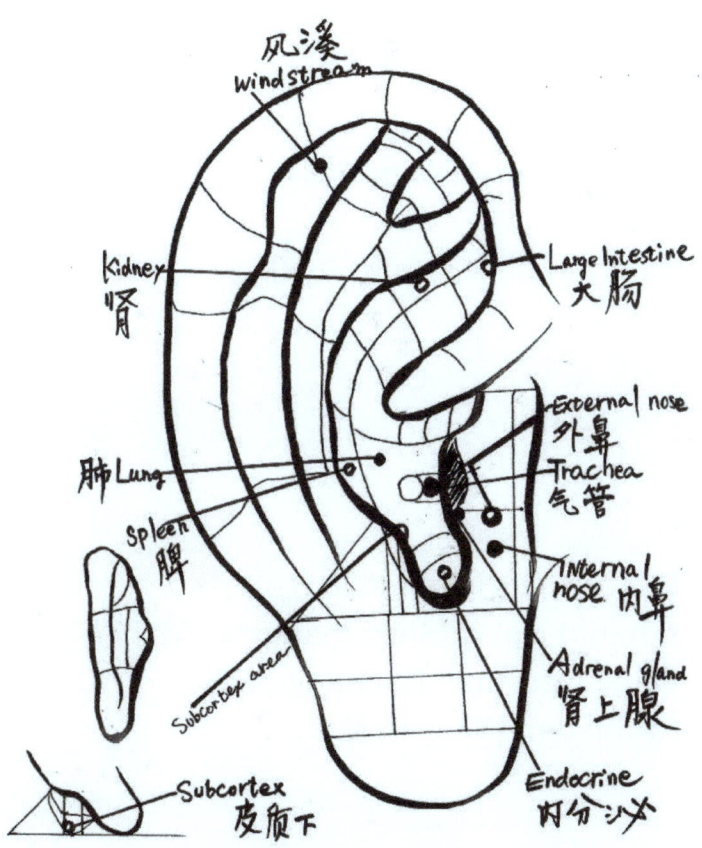

*Subcortex (Pizhixia 皮质下)... covered
*Internal nose (Neibi 内鼻)... covered

(4) Chronic Rhinitis (Manxingbiyan 慢性鼻炎)

Main points

- Internal nose (Neibi 内鼻)
- Lung (Fei 肺)
- External nose (Waibi 外鼻)

Secondary points

- Endocrine (Neifenmi 内分泌)
- Adrenal gland (Shenshangxian 肾上腺)
- Large intestine (Dachang 大肠)
- Brainstem (Naogan 脑干)

(4) Chronic Rhinitis (Manxingbiyan 慢性鼻炎)

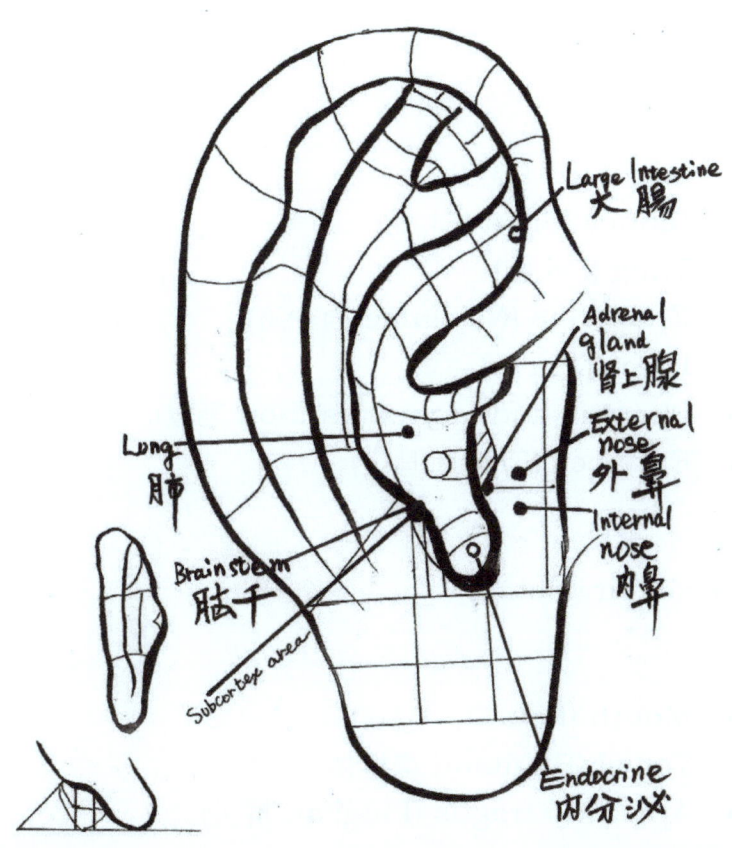

*Internal nose (Neibi 内鼻) ... covered

(5) Hoarseness (Shengyinsiya 声音嘶哑)

Main points

- Shenmen (神门)
- Kidney (Shen 肾)
- Lung (Fei 肺)
- Endocrine (Neifenme 内分泌)
- Heart (Xin 心)
- Pharynx and larynx (Yanhou 咽喉)
- Ear apex (Erjian 耳尖)

Secondary points

- Mouth (Kou 口)
- Tonsil (Biantaoti 扁桃体)
- Apex and tragus (Pingjian 屏尖)
- Large intestine (Dachang 大肠)

(5) Hoarseness (Shengyinsiya 声音嘶哑)

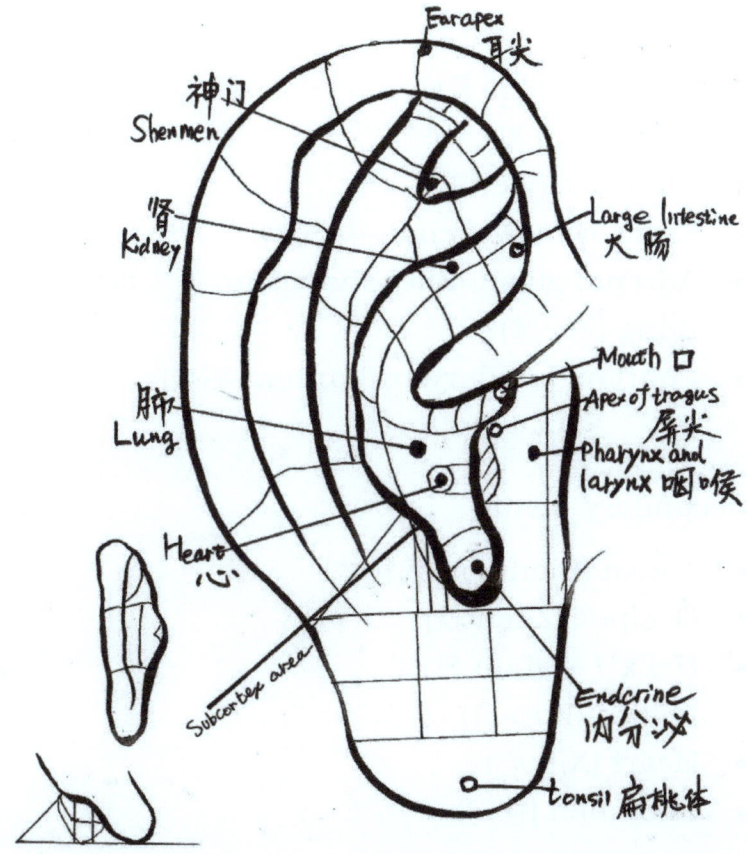

*Pharynx and larynx (Yanhou 咽喉) ...covered

(6) Pharyngitis (Yanyan 咽炎)

Main points

- Kidney (Shen 肾)
- Liver (Gan 肝)
- Stomach (Wei 胃)
- Endocrine (Neifenmi 内分泌)
- Adrenal gland (Shenshangxian 肾上腺)
- Lung (Fei 肺)
- Pharynx and larynx (Yanhou 咽喉)

Secondary points

- Tonsil (Biantaoti 扁桃体)
- Occiput (Zhen 枕)
- Helix 1-4 (Lun 轮)
- Mouth (Kou 口)
- Heart (Xin 心)
- Shenmen (神门)

(6) Pharyngitis (Yanyan 咽炎)

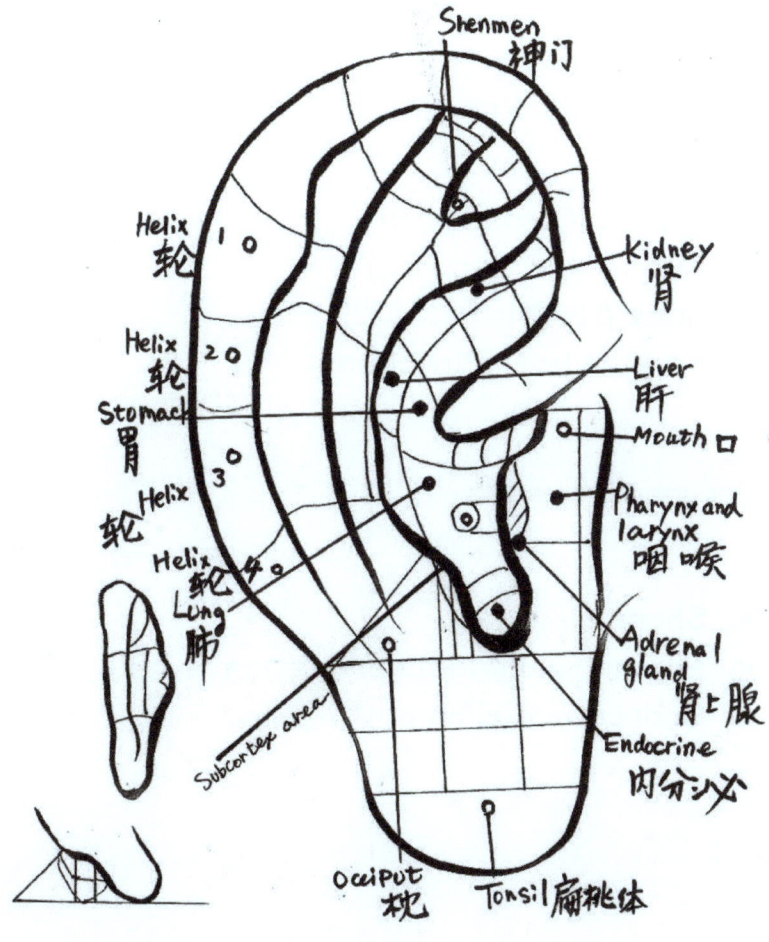

*Pharynx and larynx (Yanhou 咽喉) ···covered

(7) Acute Sore Throat (Jixingyanhouyan 急性咽喉炎)

Main points

- Tracha (Qiguan 气管)
- Ear apex (Erjian 耳尖)
- Lung (Fei 肺)
- Breathe level (Pingchuan 平喘)

Secoondary points

- Shenmen (神门)
- Adrenal gland (Shenshangxian 肾上腺)
- Endocrine (Neifenmi 内分泌)

(7) Acute Sore Throat (Jixingyanhouyan 急性咽喉炎)

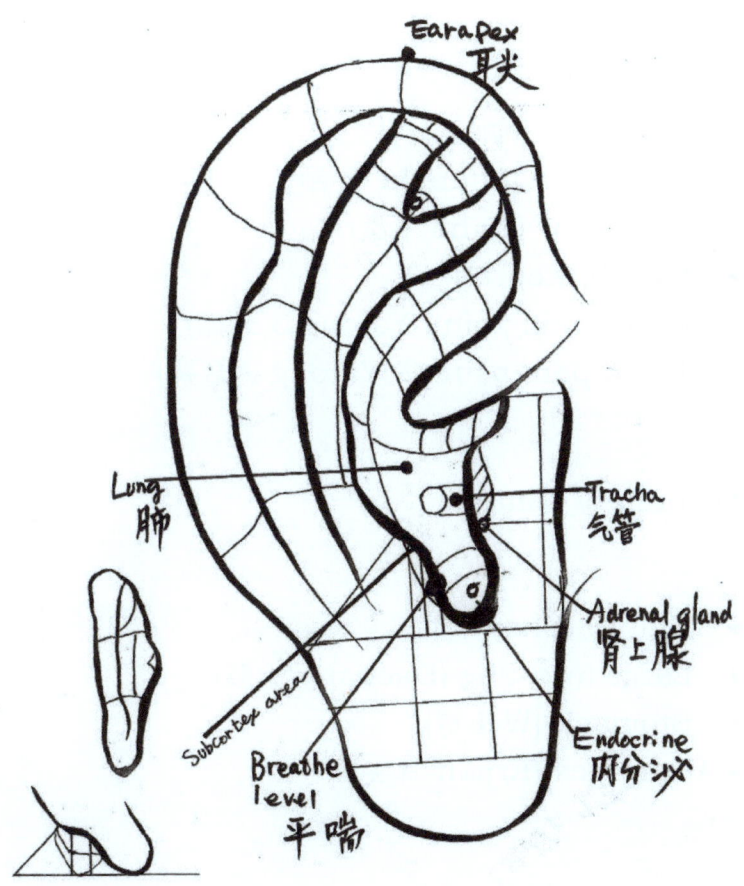

(8) Tooth ache (Yatong 牙痛)

Main points

- Shenmen (神门)
- Upper jaw (Shanghe 上颌)
- Down jaw (xiahe 下颌)
- Mouth (Kou 口)
- Tooth pain point (Yatong 3 牙痛)
- Tooth pain point 2 (Yatong 2 牙痛)

Secondary points

- Kidney (Shen 肾)
- Large intestine (Dachang 大肠)
- Stomach (Wei 胃)
- Ear apex (Erjian 耳尖)

(8) Tooth ache (Yatong 牙痛)

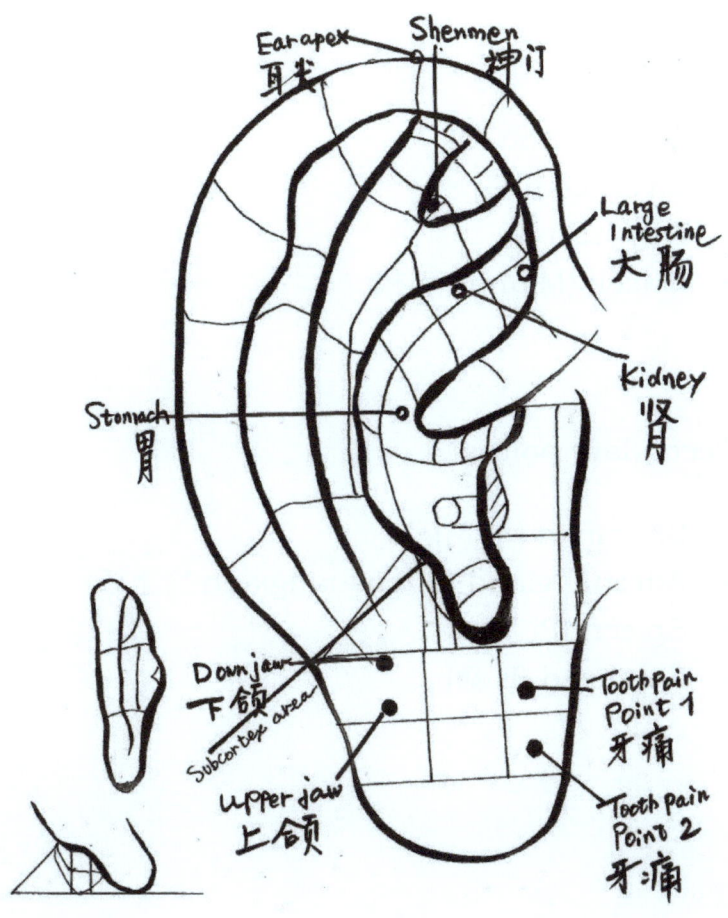

Earapex 耳尖
Shenmen 神门
Large Intestine 大肠
Kidney 肾
Stomach 胃
Down jaw 下颌
Subcortex area
Upper jaw 上颌
Tooth pain Point 1 牙痛
Tooth pain Point 2 牙痛

(9) Facial Paralysis (Miantan 面瘫)

Main points

- Mouth (Kou 口)
- Liver (Gan 肝)
- Eye (Yan 眼)
- Cheek (Mianjia 面颊)

Secondary points

- Shenmen (神门)
- Adrenal gland (Shenshangxian 肾上腺)
- Spleen (Pi 脾)
- Forehead (E 额)

(9) Facial Paralysis (Miantan 面瘫)

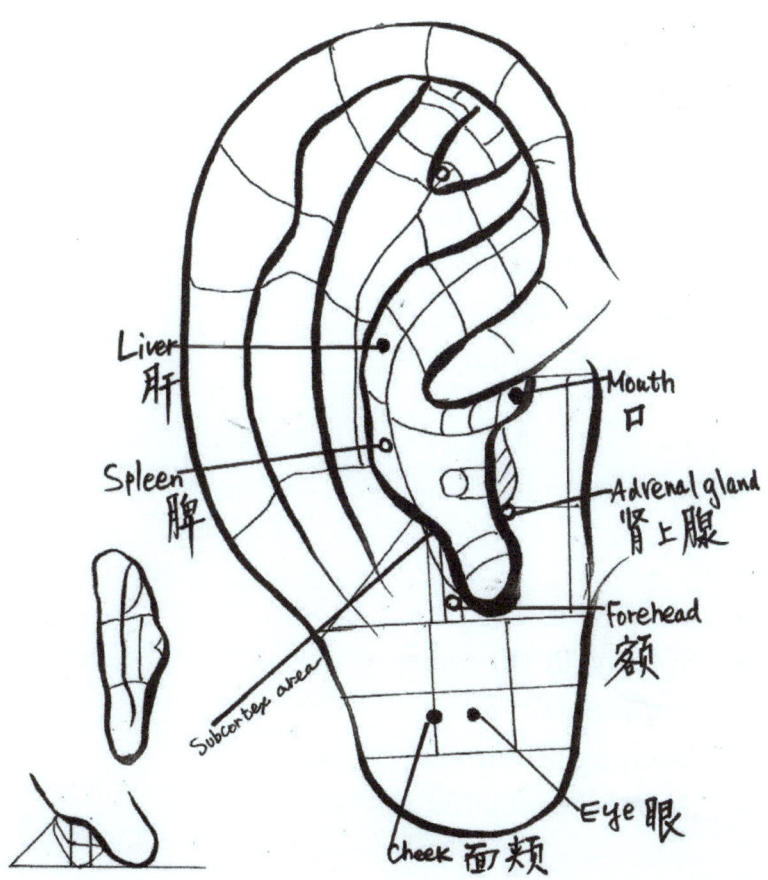

(10) Facial Spasm (Mianbujingluan 面部痉挛)

Main points

- Shenmen (神门)
- Mouth (Kou 口)
- Eye (Yan 眼)
- Cheek (Mianjia 面颊)

Secondary points

- Liver (Gan 肝)
- Spleen (Pi 脾)
- Temple (Nie 颞)
- Occiput (Zhen 枕)
- Subcortex (Pizhixia 皮质下)

(10) Facial Spasm (Mianbujingluan 面部痉挛)

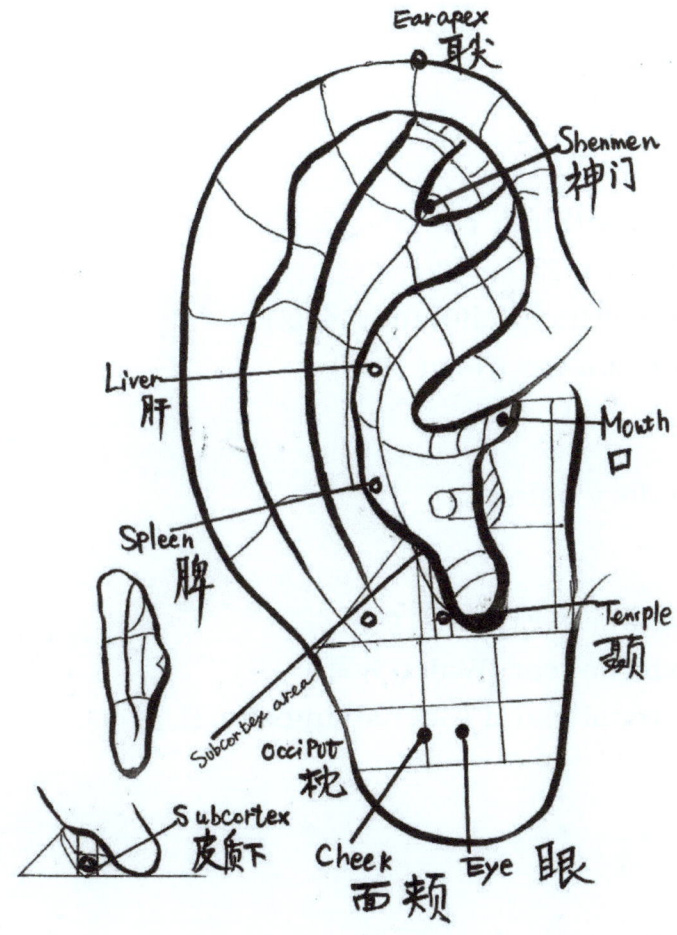

*Subcortex (Pizhixia 皮质下) ... covered

(11) Otitis Media (Zhongeryan 中耳炎)

Main points

- Kidney (Shen 肾)
- Occiput (Zhen 枕)
- Endocrine (Neifenmi 内分泌)
- Internal ear (Neier 内耳)

Secondary points

- Ear apex (Erjian 耳尖)
- External ear (Waier 外耳)
- Adrenal gland (Shenshangxian 肾上腺)

(11) Otitis Media (Zhongeryan 中耳炎)

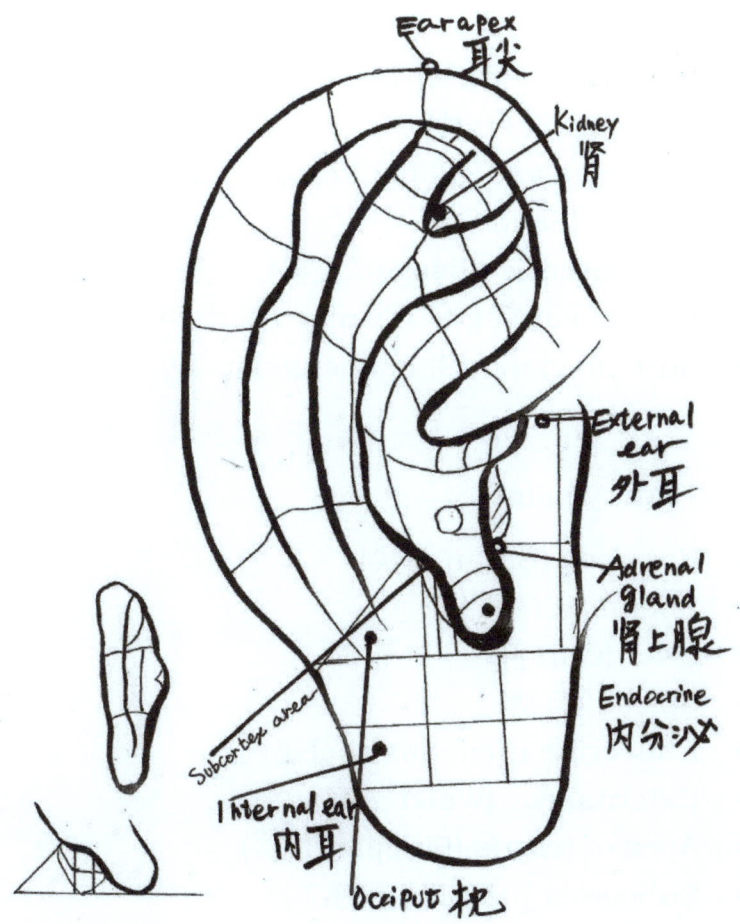

(12) Tinnitus (Erming 耳鸣)

Main points

- Internal ear (Neier 内耳)
- Occiput (Zhen 枕)
- Pancreas and gallbladder (Yidan 胰胆)
- Kidney (Shen 肾)
- Sympathesis (Jiaogan 交感)
- Root of ear vagus (Ermigen 耳迷根)
- Adrenal gland (Shenshangxian 肾上腺)

Secondary points

- Ear apex (Erjian 耳尖)
- Shenmen (神门)
- Liver (Gan 肝)
- Spleen (Pi 脾)
- Endocrine (Neifenmi 内分泌)
- External ear (Waier 外耳)
- Apex of tragus (Pingjian 屏尖)
- Subcortex (Pizhixia 皮质下)

(12) Tinnitus (Erming 耳鸣)

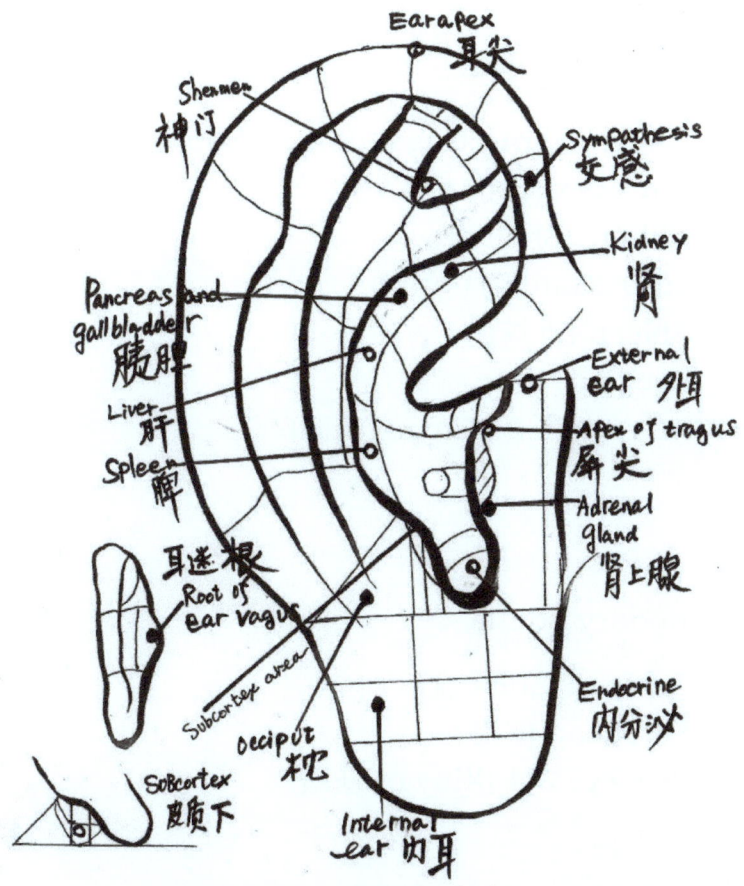

*Sympathesis (Jiaogan 交感) … covered
*Subcortex (Pizhixia 皮质下) …covered

(13) Myopia (Jinshi 近视)

Main points

- Posterior intertragal (Pinjianhou 屏间后)
- Ear apex (Erjian 耳尖)
- Kidney (Shen 肾)
- Liver (Gan 肝)
- Spleen (Pi 脾)
- Eye (Yan 眼)
- New eye 1.2 (Xinyan 新眼)

Secondary points

- Occiput (Zhen 枕)
- Forehead (E 额)
- New eye 3.4 (Xinyan 新眼)

(13) Myopia (Jinshi 近视)

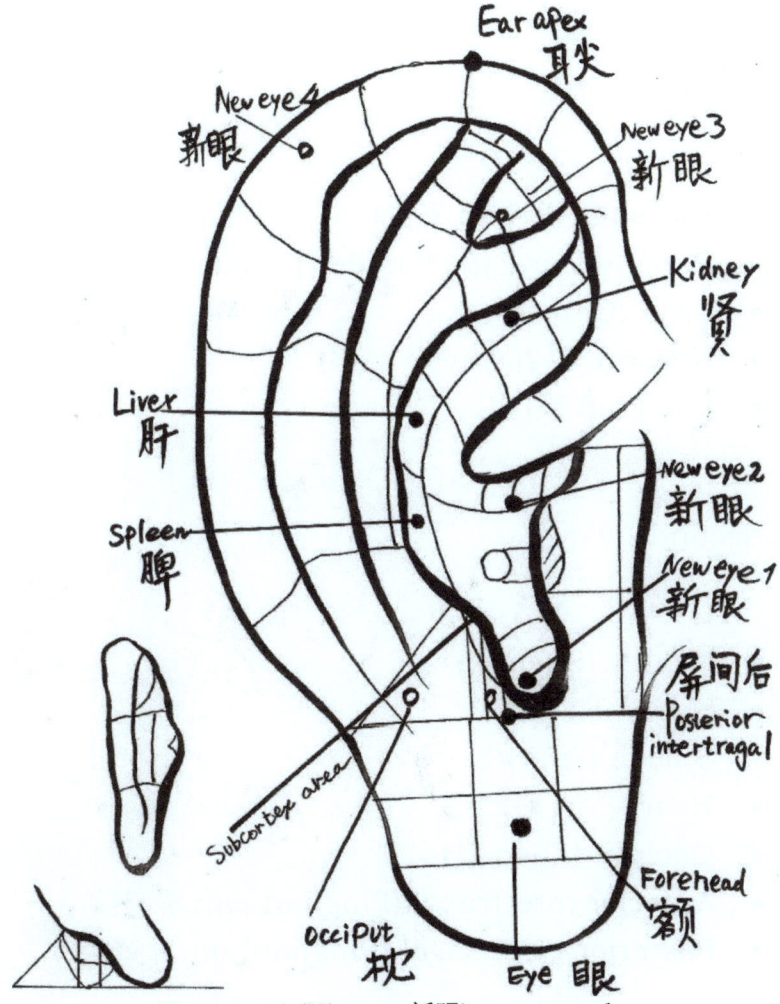

New eye 4 (Xinyan 新眼) … covered

(14) Glaucoma (Qingguangyan 青光眼)

Main points

- Ear apex (Erjian 耳尖)
- Pancreas and gallbladder (Yidan 胰胆)
- Liver (Gan 肝)
- New eye 1-2(Xinyan 新眼)
- Eye (Yan 眼)

Secondary eye

- Kidney (Shen 肾)
- Shenmen (神门)
- Spleen (Pi 脾)
- Heart (Xin 心)
- Occiput (Zhen 枕)
- Anterior intertragal (Pingjianqian 屏间前)
- Posterior intertragal (Pingjianhou 屏间后)

(14) Glaucoma (Qingguangyan 青光眼)

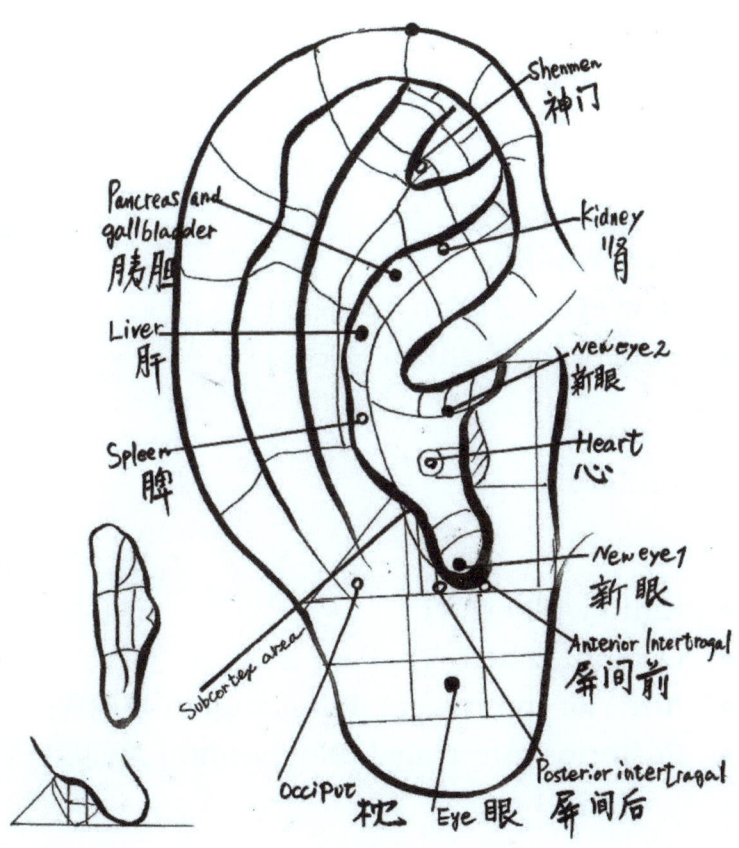

(15) Optic Atrophy (Shishenjing weisuo 视神经萎缩)

Main points

- Liver (Gan 肝)
- Eye (Yan 眼)
- New eye 1-2 (Xonyan 新眼)
- Subcortex (Pizhixia 皮质下)

Secondary points

- Kidney (Shen 肾)
- Occiput (Zhen 枕)
- Anterior intertragal (Pingjianqian 屏间前)
- Posterior intertragal (Pingjianhou 屏间后)

(15) Optic Atrophy (Shishenjing weisuo 视神经萎缩)

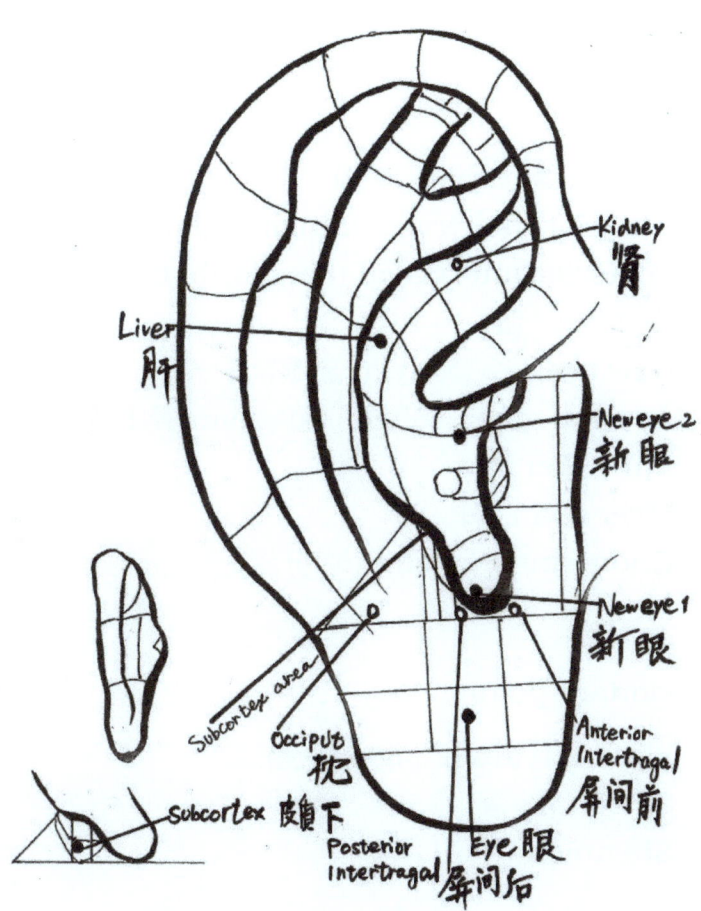

Kidney 肾

Liver 肝

New eye 2 新眼

New eye 1 新眼

Subcortex area

Occiput 枕

Anterior Intertragal 屏间前

Subcortex 颞下

Posterior Intertragal 屏间后

Eye 眼

* Subcortex (Pizhixia 皮质下)… covered

(16) Acute Conjunctivitis (Jixingjiemoyan 急性结膜炎)

Main points

- Ear apex (Erjian 耳尖)
- Anterior intertragal (Pingjianqian 屏间前)
- Posterior intertragal (Pingjianhou 屏间后)
- Eye (Yan 眼)
- New eye 1-2 (Xinyan 新眼)
- Adrenal gland (Shenshangxian 肾上腺)
- Lung (Fei 肺)
- Liver (Gan 肝)
- Endocrine (Neifenmi 内分泌)

Secondary points

- Wind stream (Fengxi 风溪)
- Spleen (Pi 脾)
- Shenmen (神门)

(16) Acute Conjunctivitis (Jixingjiemoyan 急性结膜炎)

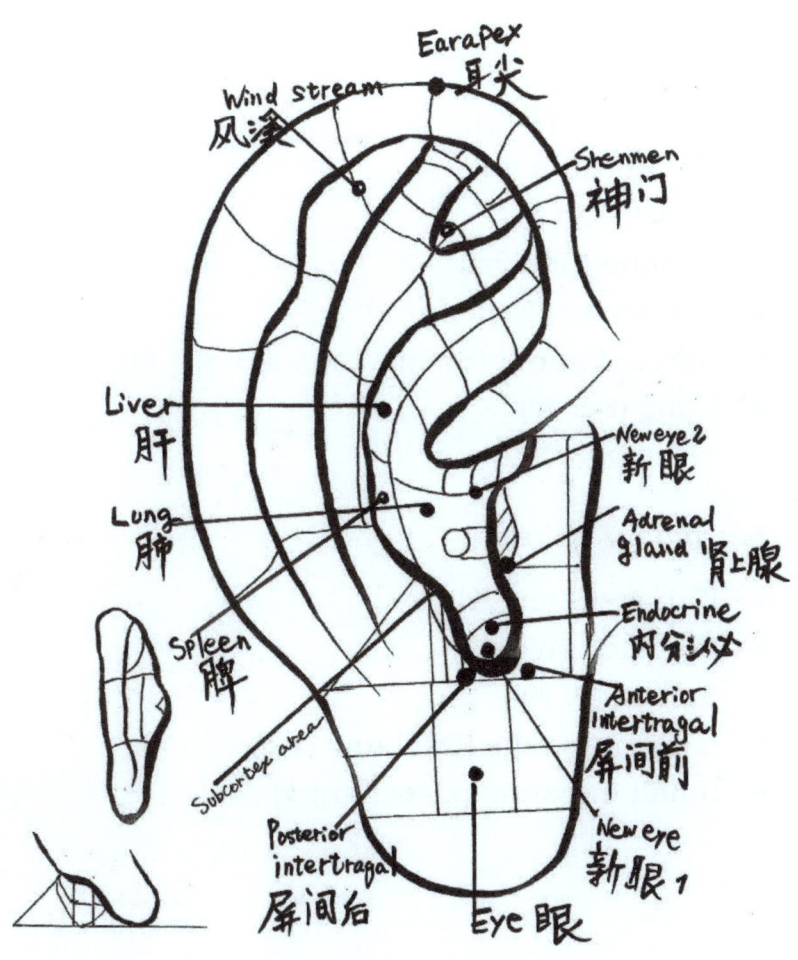

(17) Mouth ulcer (Kouqiangkuiyang 口腔溃疡)

Main points

- Shenmen (神门)
- Mouth (Kou 口)
- Heart (Xin 心)
- Tongue (She 舌)
- Endocrine (Neifenmi 内分泌)
- Adrenal gland (Shenshangxian 肾上腺)
- Lung (Fei 肺)

Secondary points

- Kidney (Shen 肾)
- Stomach (Wei 胃)
- Spleen (Pi 脾)
- Large intestine (Dachang 大肠)
- Small intestine (xiaochang 小肠)

(17) Mouth ulcer (Kouqiangkuiyang 口腔溃疡)

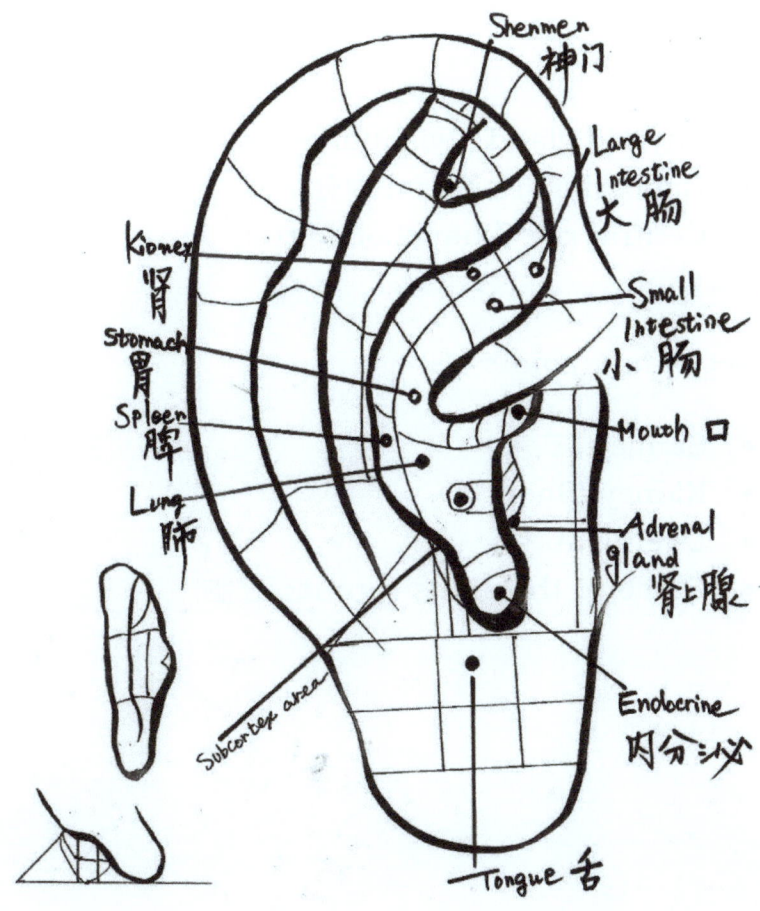

(18) Goiter (Jiazhuangxianzhong 甲状腺肿)

Main points

- Thyroid gland (Jiazhuangxian 甲状腺)
- Endocrine (Neifenmi 内分泌)
- Central rim (Yuanzhong 缘中)

Secondary points

- Sanjiao (三焦)
- Kidney (Shen 肾)
- Liver (Gan 肝)
- Cerebral thalamus (Qiunao 丘脑)

(18) Goiter (Jiazhuangxianzhong 甲状腺肿)

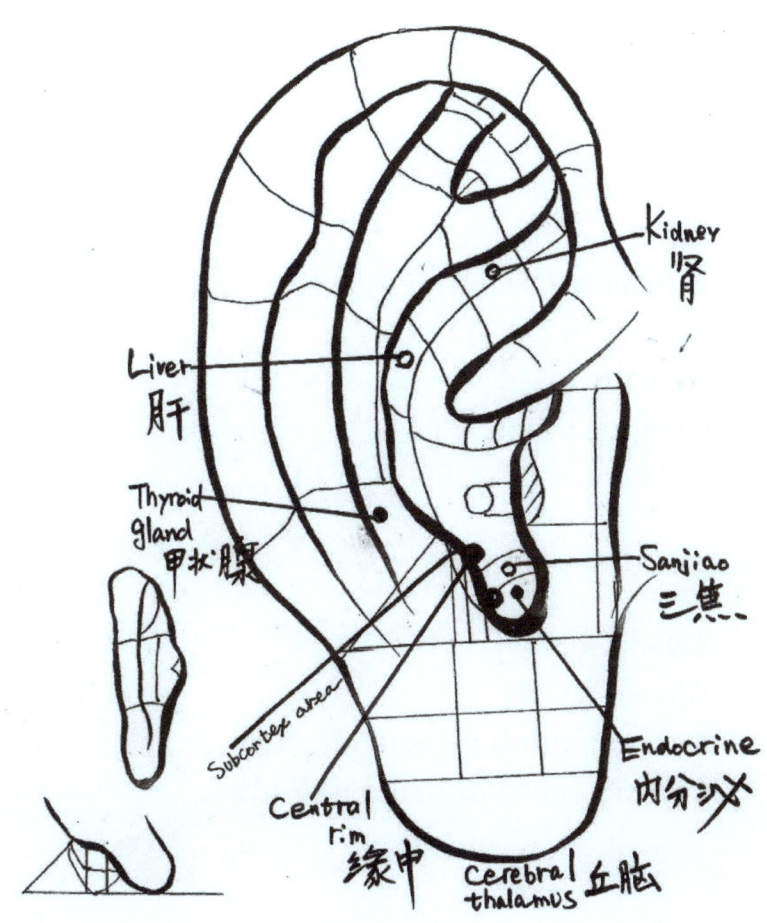

CHAPTER 5. Dermatological Diseases

(1) Psoriasis (Yinxiebing 银屑病)

Main points

- Ear apex (Erjian 耳尖)
- Lung (Fei 肺)
- Endcrine (Neifenmi 内分泌)
- Shenmen (神门)
- Heart (Xin 心)
- Occiput (Zhen 枕)
- Subcortex (Pizhixia 皮质下)

Supporting points

- Liver (Gan 肝)
- Spleen (Pi 脾)
- Adrenal gland (Shenshangxian 肾上腺)
- Central rim (Yuanzhong 缘中)

(1) Psoriasis (Yinxiebing 银屑病)

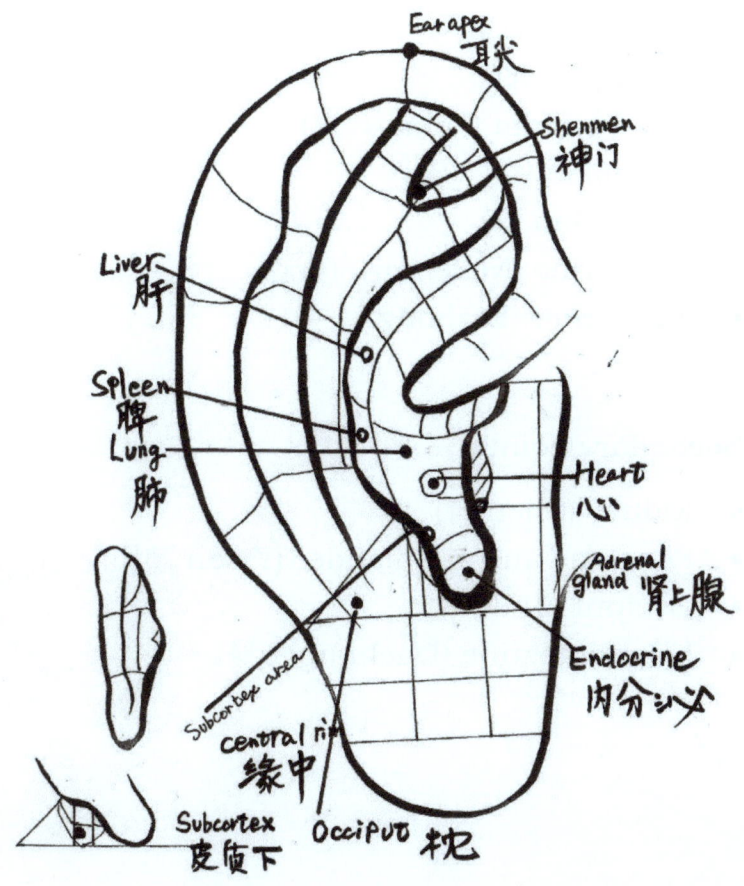

*Subcortex (Pizhixia 皮质下)... covered

(2) Pruritus (Saoyang 瘙痒)

Main points

- Lung (Fei 肺)
- Wind stream (Fenxi 风溪)
- Shenmen (神门)
- Liver (Gan 肝)
- Endocrine (Neifenmi 内分泌)
- Ear center (Erzhong 耳中)

Secondary points

- Kidney (Shen 肾)
- Pancreas and gallbladder (Yidan 胰胆)
- Occiput (Zhen 枕)
- Large intestine (Dachang 大肠)

(2) Pruritus (Saoyang 瘙痒)

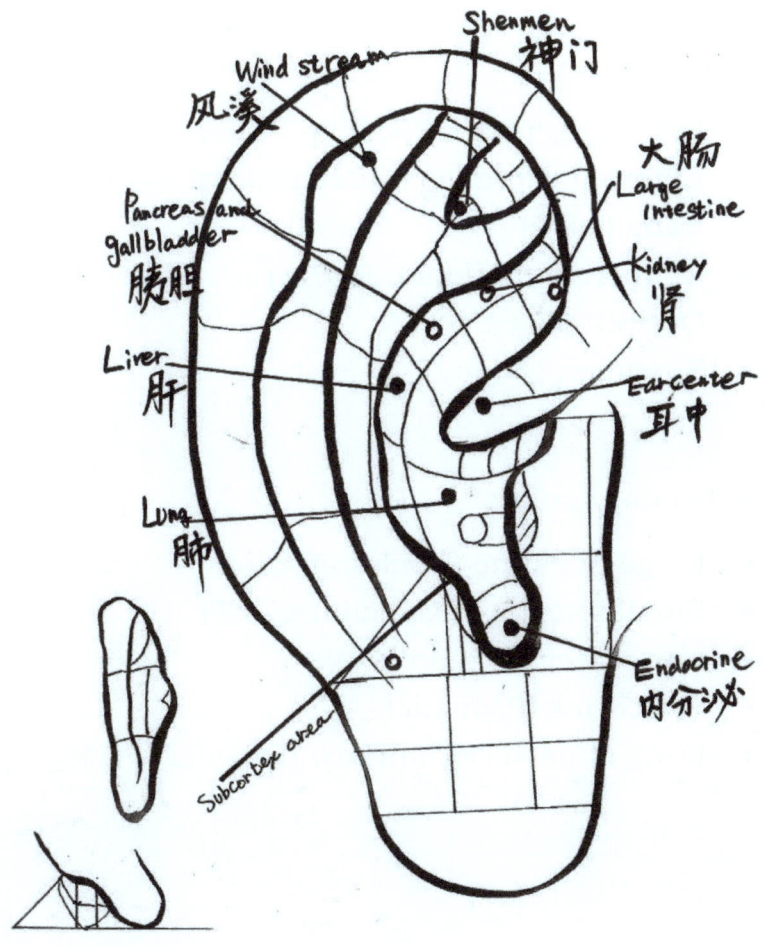

(3) Pruritus Vulvae (Waiyinsaoyang 外阴瘙痒)

Main points

- Internal genitals (Neizhiqi 内殖器)
- External genitals (Waishengzhiqi 外生殖器)
- Lung (fei 肺)
- Endocrine (Neifenmi 内分泌)
- Occiput (Zhen 枕)
- Shenmen (神门)

Secondary points

- Large intestine (Dachang 大肠)
- Small intestine (Xiaochang 小肠)
- Ear center (Erzhon 耳中)
- Subcortex (Pizhixia 皮质下)
- Lung of posterior surface (Erbeifei 耳背肺)

(3) Pruritus Vulvae (Waiyinsaoyang 外阴瘙痒)

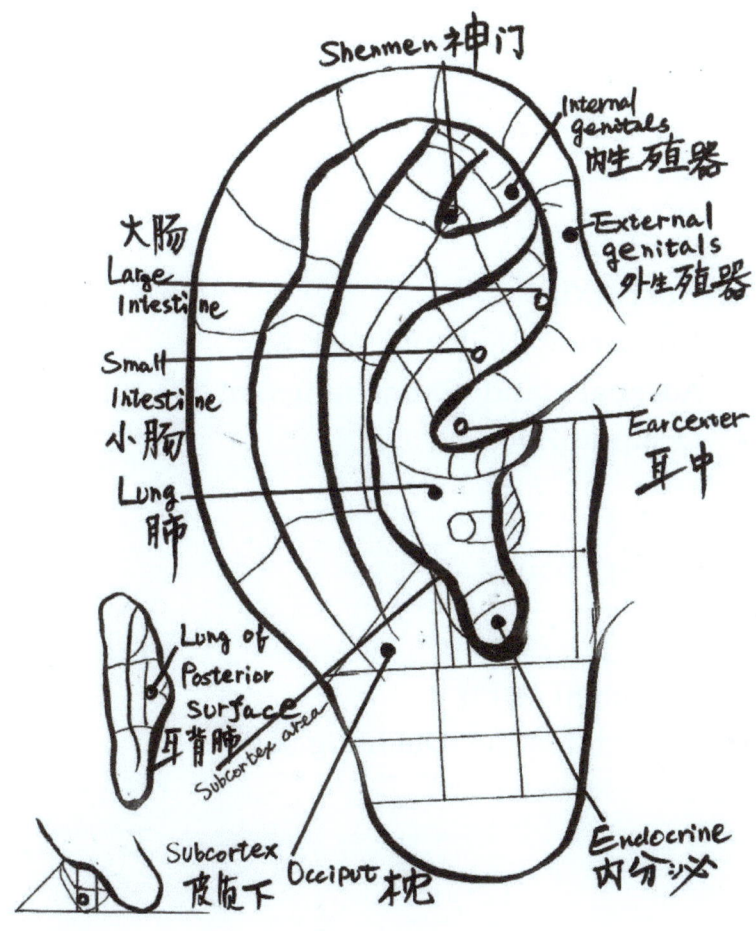

*Subcortex (Pizhixia 皮质下) … covered

(4) Seborrheic Dermatitis (Zhiyixingpiyan 脂溢性皮炎)

Main points

- Lung (Fei 肺)
- Heart (Xin 心)
- Endocrine (Neifenmi 内分泌)
- Adrenal gland (Shenshangxian 肾上腺)
- Occiput (Zhen 枕)

Secondary points

- Shenmen (神门)
- Large intestine (Dachang 大肠)

(4) Seborrheic Dermatitis (Zhiyixingpiyan 脂溢性皮炎)

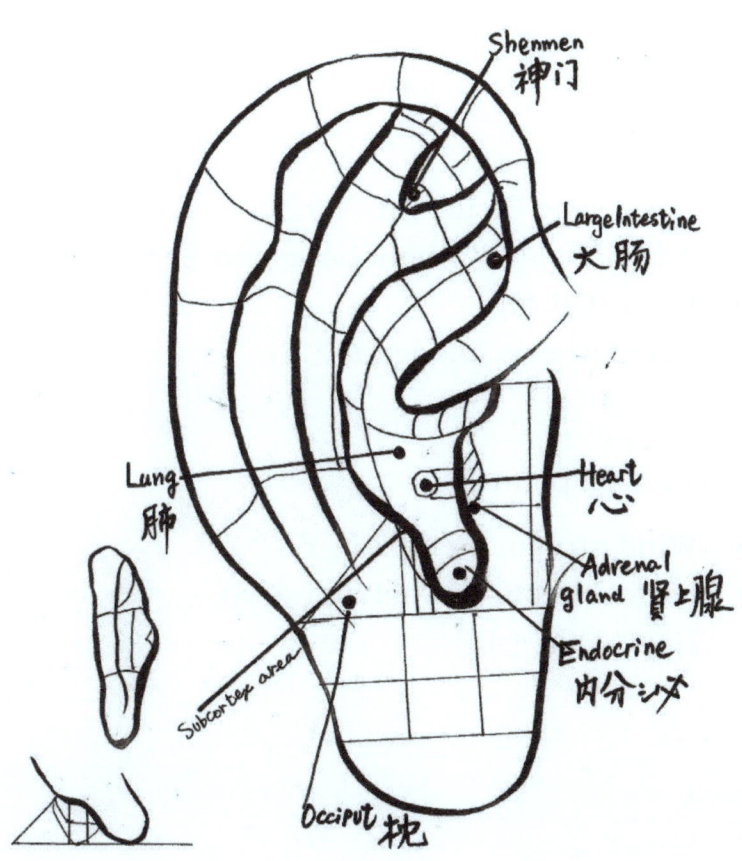

(5) Allergic Dermatitis (Guominxingpiyan 过敏性皮炎)

Main points

- Endocrine (Neifenmi 内分泌)
- Adrenal gland (Shenshangxian 肾上腺)
- Lung (Fei 肺)
- Sympathesis (Jiaogan 交感)

Secondary points

- Wind stream (Fengxi 风溪)
- Large intestine (Dachang 大肠)
- Heart (Xin 心)

(5) Allergic Dermatitis (Guominxingpiyan 过敏性皮炎)

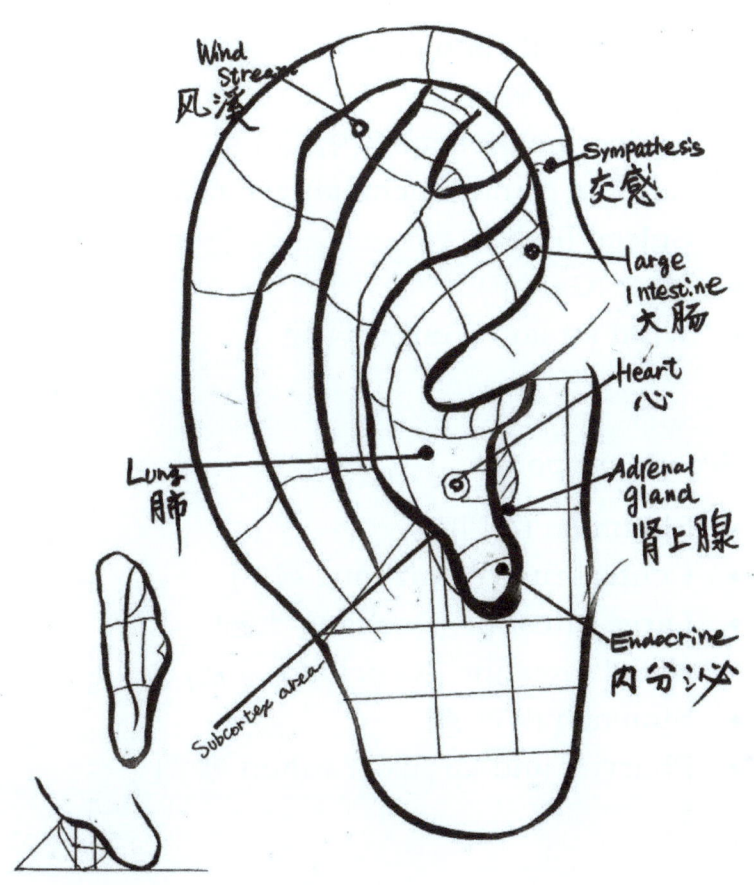

(6) Urticaria (Xunmazhen 荨麻疹)

Main points

- Ear apex (Erjian 耳尖)
- Lung (Fei 肺)
- Endocrine (Neifenmi 内分泌)
- Adrenal gland (Shenshangxian 肾上腺)
- Spleen (Pi 脾)
- Liver (Gan 肝)
- Wind stream (Fengxi 风溪)

Secondary points

- Shenmen (神门)
- Central rim (Yuanzhong 缘中)
- Large intestine (Dachang 大肠)
- Small intestine (Xiaochang 小肠)
- Stomach (Wei 胃)
- Pharynx and larynx (Yanhou 咽喉)

(6) Urticaria (Xunmazhen 荨麻疹)

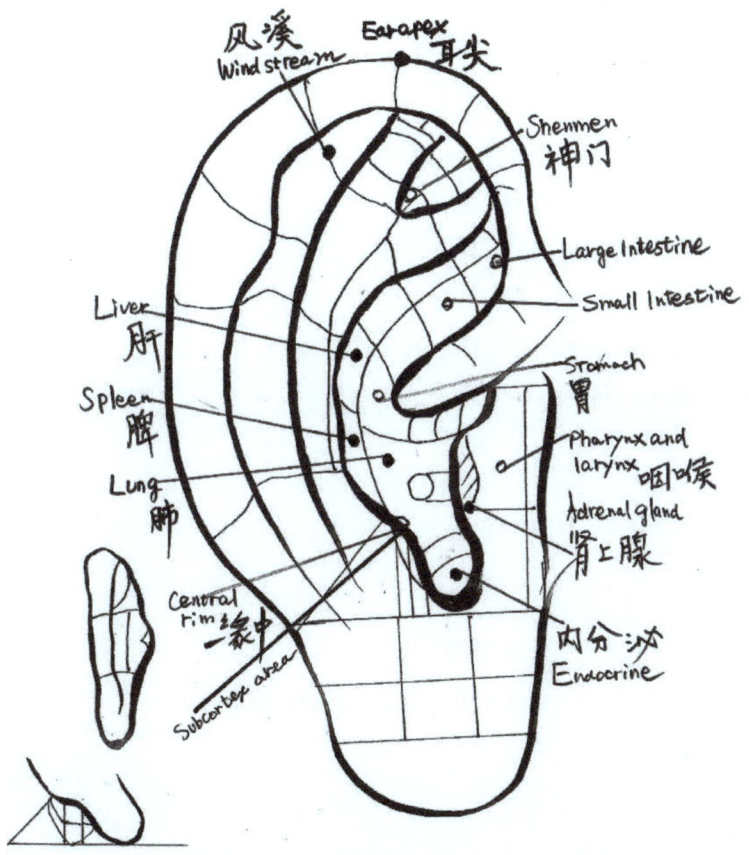

*Pharynx and larynx (Yanhou 咽喉) ...covered

(7) Herpes Zoster (Daizhuangpaozhen 带状疱疹)

Main points

- Ear apex (Erjian 耳尖)
- Kidney (Shen 肾)
- Shenmen (神门)
- Liver (Gan 肝)
- Endocrine (Neifenmi 内分泌)
- Subcortex (Pizhixia 皮质下)

Secondary points

- Occiput (Zhen 枕)
- Anterior earlobe (Chuiqian 垂前)

(7) Herpes Zoster (Daizhuangpaozhen 带状疱疹)

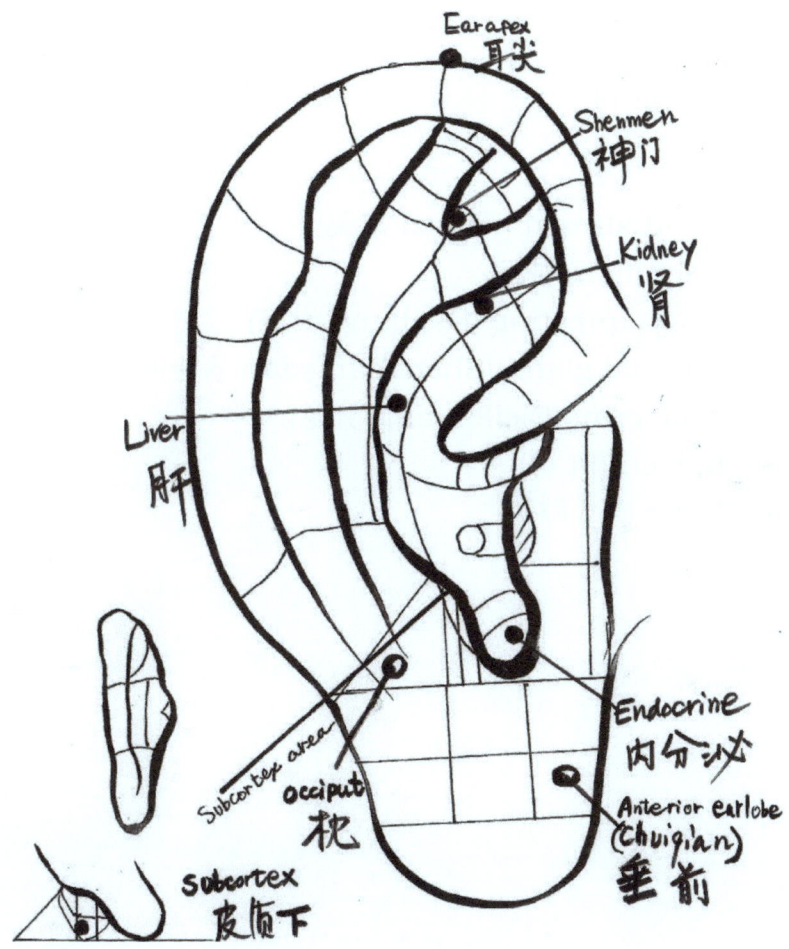

*Subcortex (Pizhixia 皮质下) … covered

(8) Eczema (Shizhen 湿疹)

Main points

- Wind stream (Fengxi 风溪)
- Shenmen (神门)
- Large intestine (Dachang 大肠)
- Adrenal gland (Shenshangxian 肾上腺)
- Endocrine (Neifenmi 内分泌)
- Spleen (Pi 脾)
- Lung (Fei 肺)

(8) Eczema (Shizhen 湿疹)

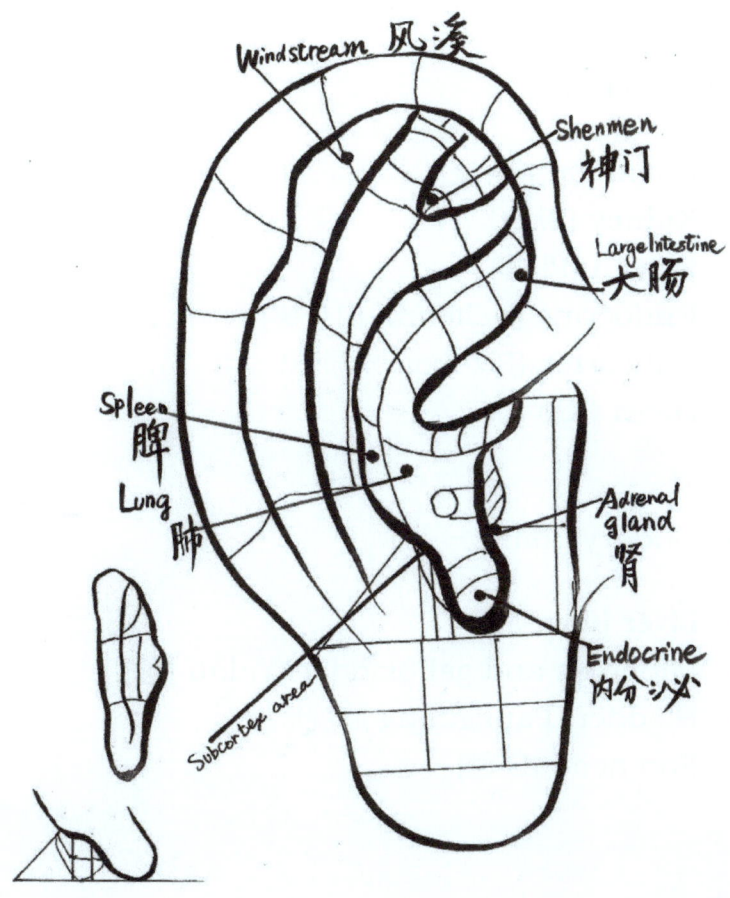

(9) Lose hair (Tuofa 脱发)

Main points

- Shenmen (神门)
- Kidney (Shen 肾)
- Spleen (Pi 脾)
- Endocrine (Neifenmi 内分泌)
- Subcortex (Pizhixia 皮质下)
- Heart (Xin 心)

Secondary points

- Liver (Gan 肝)
- Pancreas and gallbladder (Yidan 胰胆)
- Bladder (Pangguang 膀胱)
- Forehead (E 额)

(9) Lose hair (Tuofa 脱发)

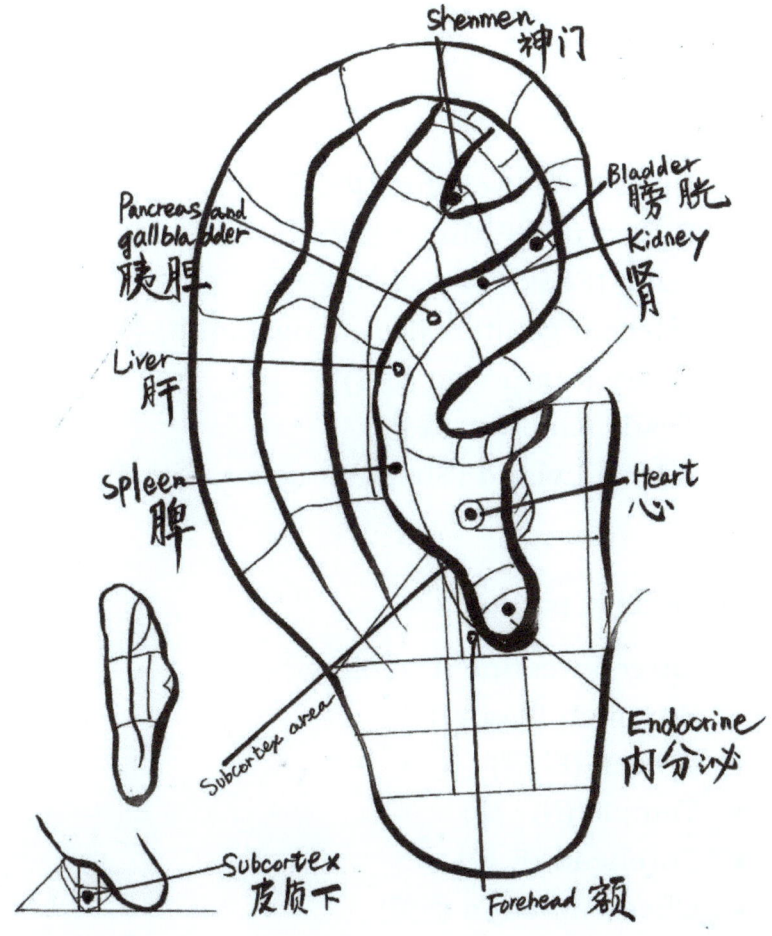

*Subcortex (Pizhixia 皮质下)··· covered

CHAPTER 6. Cosmetic Acupuncture

(1) Acne (Cuochuang 痤疮)

Main points

- Endocrine (Neifenmi 内分泌)
- Subcortex (Pizhixia 皮质下)
- Lung (Fei 肺)
- Internal genitals (Neishengzhiqi 内生殖器)
- Ovary (Luanchao 卵巢)
- Testis (Gaowan 睾丸)
- Adrenal gland (Shenshangxian 肾上腺)

Secondary points

- Large intestine (Dachang 大肠)
- Stomach (Wei 胃)
- Spleen (Pi 脾)
- Temple (Nie 颞)
- Forehead (E 额)
- Cheek (Mianjia 面颊)

(1) Acne (Cuochuang 痤疮)

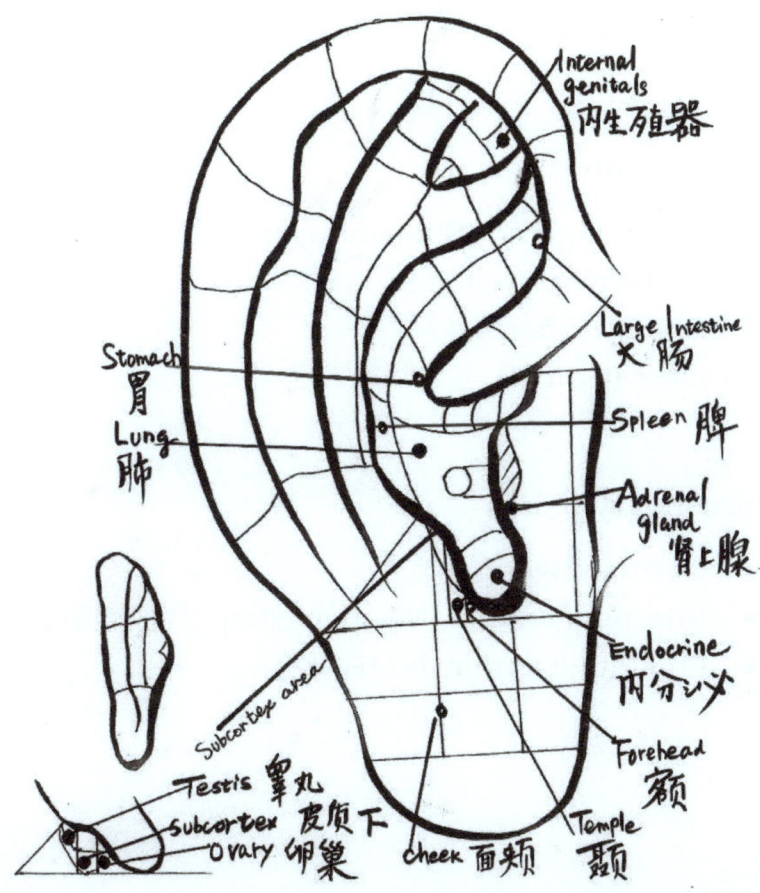

Internal genitals 内生殖器

Large Intestine 大肠

Spleen 脾

Adrenal gland 肾上腺

Endocrine 内分泌

Forehead 额

Temple 颞

cheek 面颊

Stomach 胃

Lung 肺

Subcortex area

Testis 睾丸

Subcortex 皮质下

Ovary 卵巢

*Subcortex (Pizhixia 皮质下), Testis (Gaowan 睾丸)
and Ovary (Luanchao 卵巢) …covered

(2) Chloasma, Melasma (Huangheban 黄褐斑)

Main points

- Adrenal gland (Shenshangxian 肾上腺)
- Endocrine (Neifenmi 内分泌)
- Kidney (Shen 肾)
- Liver (Gan 肝)

Secondary points

- Uterus (Zigong 子宫)
- Internal genitals (Neishengzhiqi 内生殖器)
- Prostate (Qianliexian 前列腺)

(2) Chloasma, Melasma (Huangheban 黄褐斑)

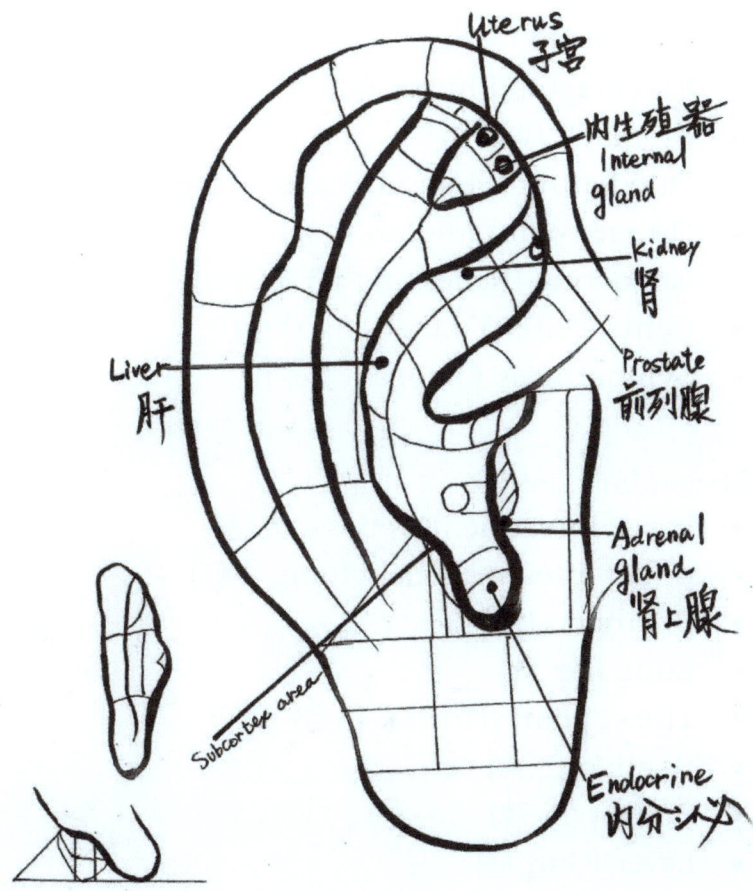

(3) Weight loss (Jianfei 减肥)

Main points
- Mouth (Kou 口)
- Esophagus (Shidao 食道)
- Stomach (Wei 胃)
- Duodenum (Shierzhichang 十二指肠)
- Hunger point (Jidian 飢点)
- Endocrine (Neifenmi 内分泌)
- Central rim (Yuanzhong 缘中)
- Sympathesis (Jiaogan 交感)

Secondary points
- Large intestine (Dachang 大肠)
- Small intestine (Xiaochang 小肠)
- Shenmen (神门)
- Lung (Fei 肺)
- Thirst point (Hedian 喝点)
- Sanjiao (三焦)
- Spleen (Pi 脾)
- Lever (Gan 肝)
- Subcortex (Pizhixia 皮质下)

(3) Weight loss (Jianfei 减肥)

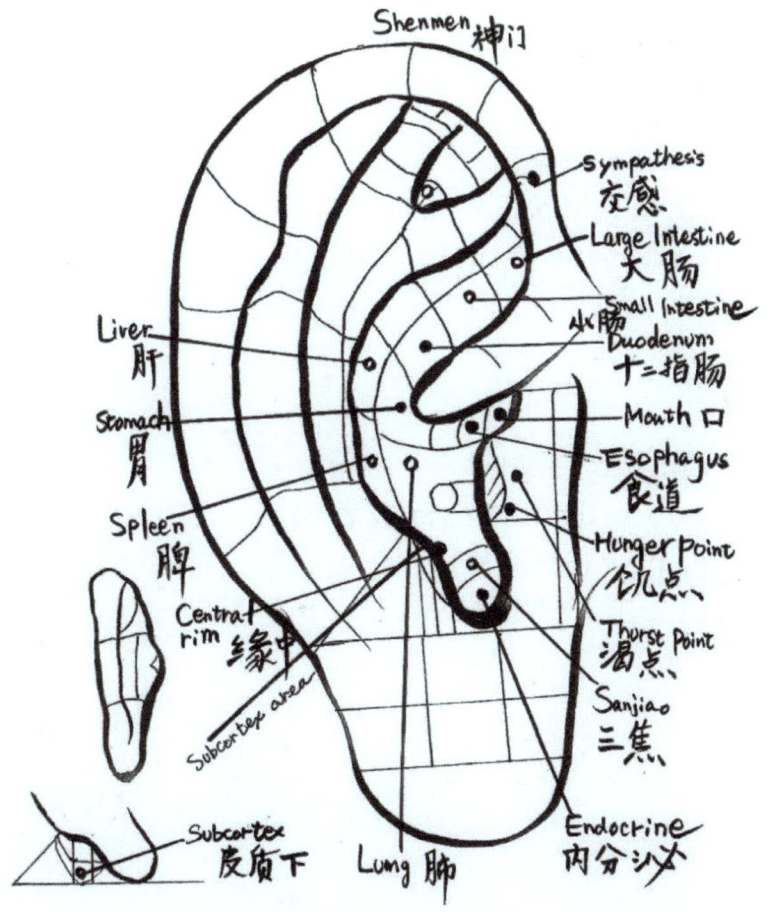

* Sympathesis (Jiaogan 交感) … covered
* Subcortex (Pizhixia 皮质下)… covered

(4) Cosmetic treatment (Meirong 美容)

Main points

- Lung (Fei 肺)
- Cheek (Mianjia 面颊)
- Endocrine (Neifenmi 内分泌)

Secondary points

- Sanjiao (三焦)
- Subcortex (Pizhixia 皮质下)
- Kidney (Shen 肾)
- Spleen (Pi 脾)

(4) Cosmetic treatment (Meirong 美容)

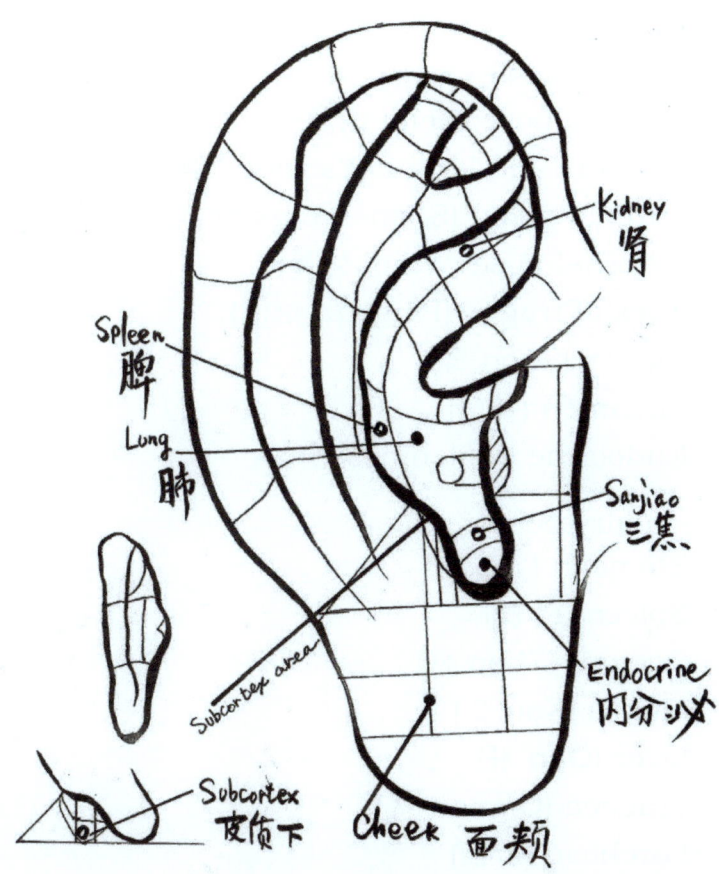

* Subcortex (Pizhixia 皮质下)... covered

CHARPTER 7. Others

(1) Cold (Ganmao 感冒)

Main points

- Lung (Fei 肺)
- Internal nose (Neibi 内鼻)
- Pharynx and larynx (Yanhou 咽喉)
- Adrenal gland (Shenshangxian 肾上腺)
- External nose (Waibi 外鼻)
- Apex of tragus (Pingjian 屏间)
- Kidney (Shen 肾)
- Shenmen (神门)
- Endocrine (Neifenmi 内分泌)

Secondary points

- Stomach (Wei 胃)
- Spleen (Pi 脾)
- Occiput (Zhen 枕)
- Mouth (Kou 口)
- Liver (Gan 肝)
- Trachea (Qiguan 气管)
- Forehead (E 额)
- Temple (Nie 聂)
- Large intestine (Dachang 大肠)
- Ear apex (Erjian 耳尖))

(1) Cold (Ganmao 感冒)

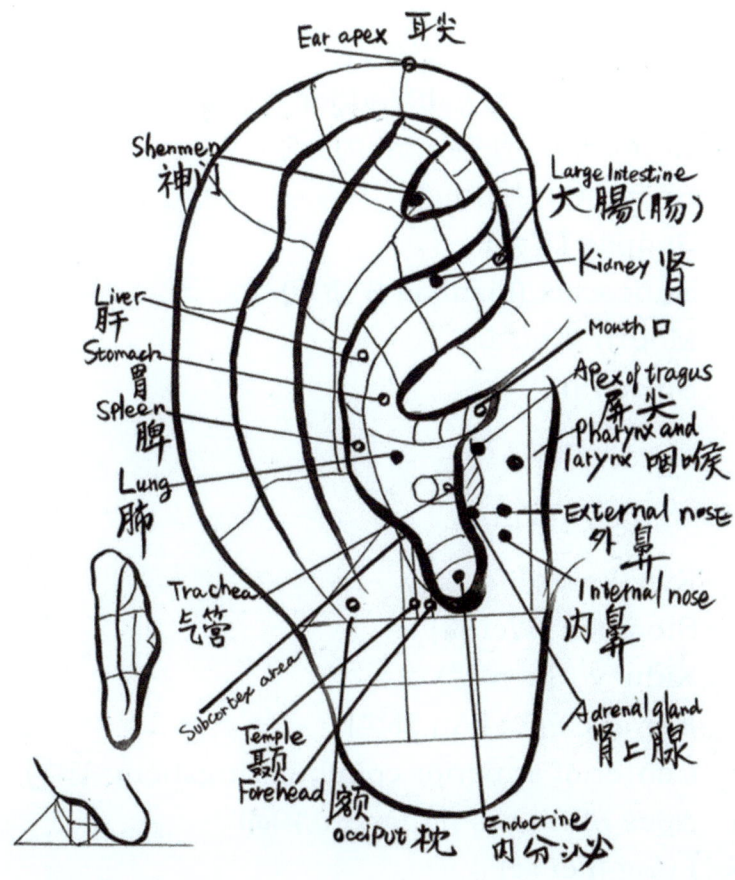

* Internal nose (Neibi 内鼻) ... covered
* Pharynx and larynx (Yanhou 咽喉) ...covered

(2) Diabetes (Tangniaobing 糖尿病)

Main points

- Pancreas and gallbladder (Yidan 胰胆)
- Endocrine (Neifenmi 内分泌)
- Shenmen (神门)
- Sanjiao (三焦)
- Subcortex (Pizhixia 皮质下)
- Mouth (Kou 口)
- Spleen (Pi 脾)

Secondary points

- Eye (Yan 眼)
- Stomach (Wei 胃)
- Kidney (Shen 肾)
- Ear apex (Er jian 耳尖)
- Center of superior concha (Tingzhong 艇中)
- Apex of tragus (Pingjian 屏间)
- Lung (Fei 肺)
- Root of ear vagus (Ermigen 耳迷根)

(2) Diabetes (Tangniaobing 糖尿病)

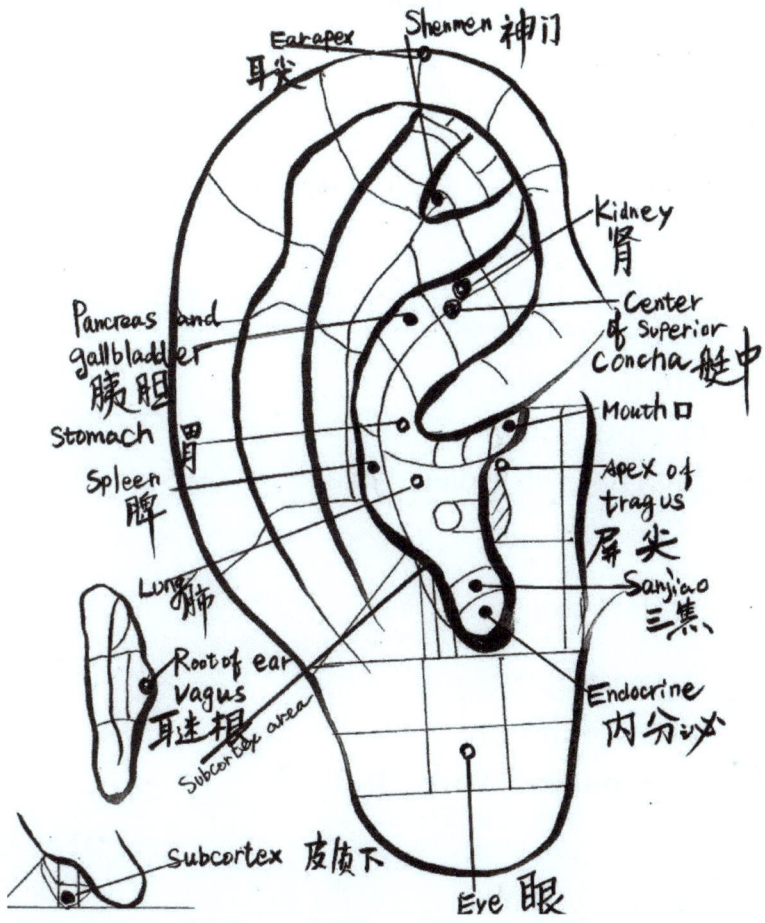

*Subcortex (Pizhixia 皮质下) …covered

(3) Car and Sea sickness (Qiche he yunchuan 汽车和晕船)

Main points

- Shenmen (神门)
- Kidney (Shen 肾)
- Stomach (Wei 胃)
- Occiput (Zhen 枕)
- Internal ear (Neier 内耳)

Secondary points

- Mouth (Kou 口)
- External ear (Waier 外耳)

(3) Car and Sea sickness (Qiche he yunchuan 汽车和晕船)

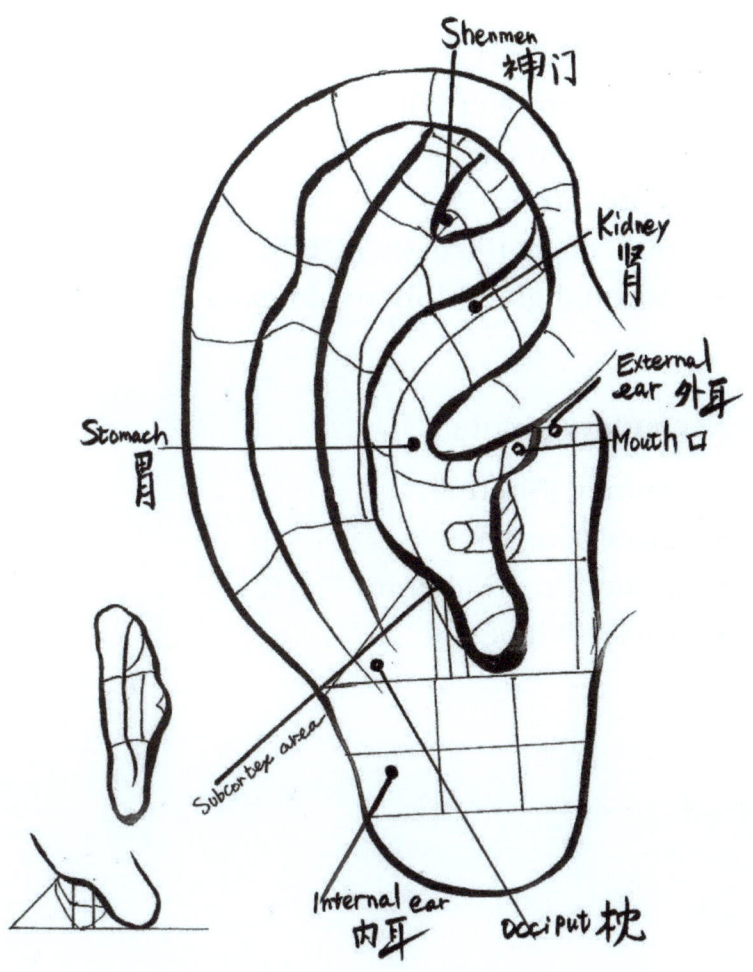

(4) Give up smoking (Jieyan 戒烟)

Main points

- Lung (Fei 肺)
- Stomach (Wei 胃)
- Shenmen (神门)
- Mouth (Kou 口)
- Subcortex (Pizhixia 皮质下)
- Adrenal gland (Shenshangxian 肾上腺)

Secondary points

- Kidney (Shen 肾)
- Liver (Gan 肝)
- Endocrine (Neifenmi 内分泌)
- Heart (Xin 心)

(4) Give up smoking (Jieyan 戒烟)

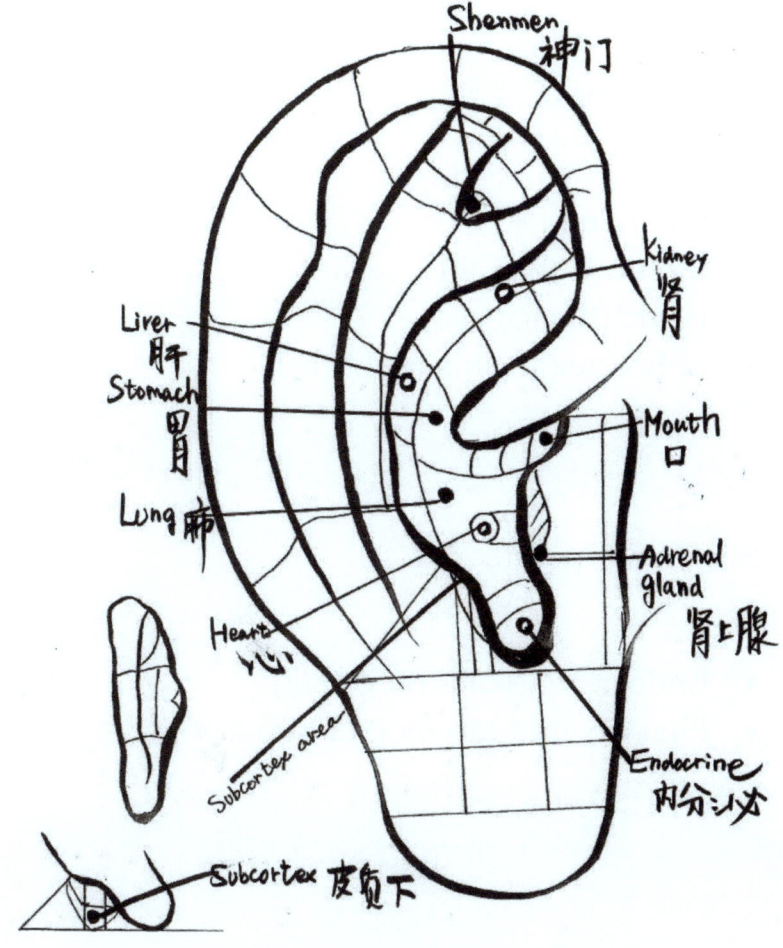

*Subcortex (Pizhixia 皮质下) …covered

(5) Stop drinking (Tinzhihejiu 停止喝酒)

Main points

- Shenmen (神门)
- Stomach (Wei 胃)
- Heart (Xin 心)
- Subcortex (Pizhixia 皮质下)

Secondary points

- Endocrine (Neifenmi 内分泌)
- Pharynx and larynx (Yanhou 咽喉)

(5) Stop drinking (Tinzhihejiu 停止喝酒)

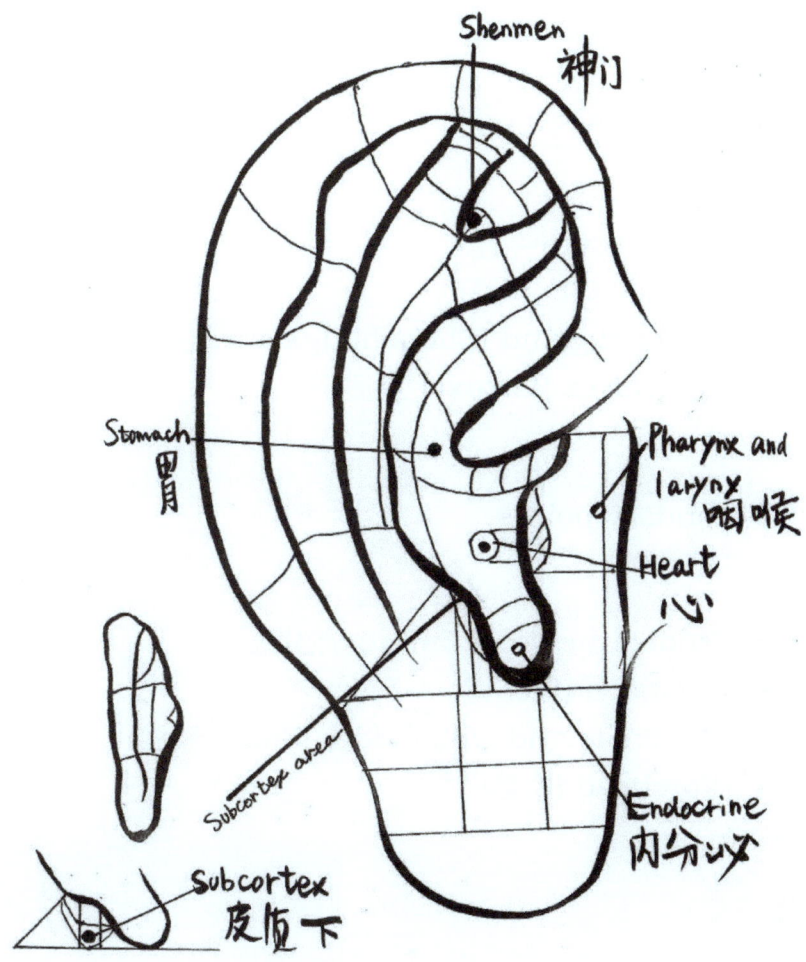

*Subcortex (Pizhixia 皮质下) ...covered

(6) Fatigue (Pilao 疲劳)

Main points

- Shenmen (神门)
- Kidney (Shen 肾)
- Adrenal gland (Shenshangxian 肾上腺)
- Subcortex (Pizhixia 皮质下)

Secondary points

- Endocrine (Neifenmi 内分泌)
- Stomach (Wei 胃)
- Pancreas and gallbladder (Yidan 胰胆)
- Forehead (E 额)

(6) Fatigue (Pilao 疲劳)

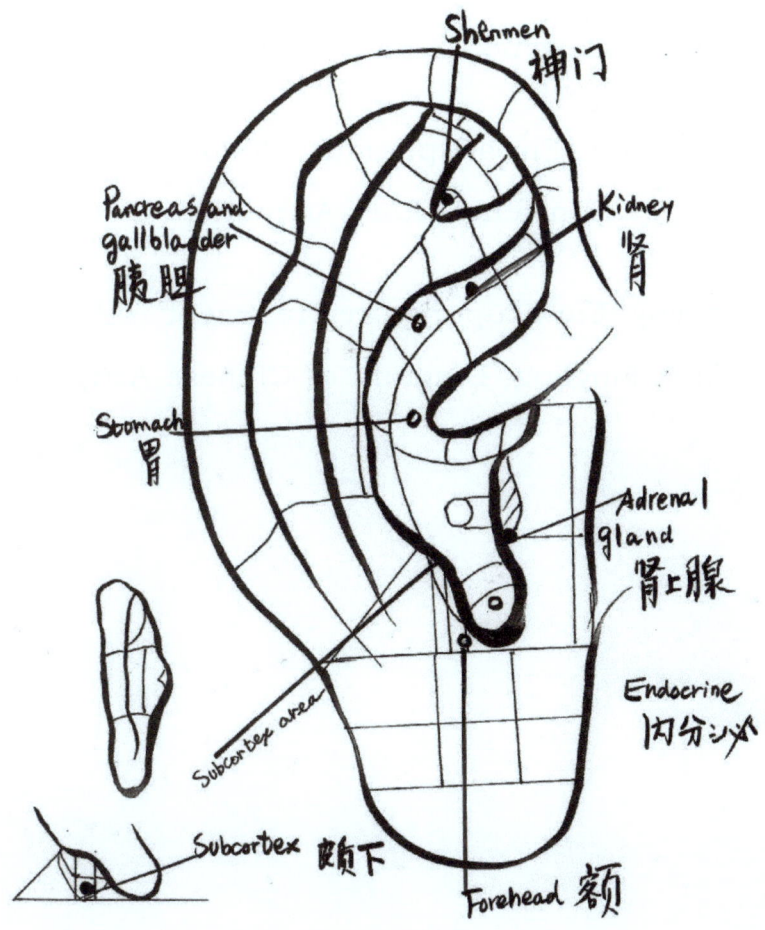

*Subcortex (Pizhixia 皮质下)... covered

References 参考文献

1. Deng Liangyue, Chinese Acupuncture and Moxibution 1987.

2. Zhu Jiang, Ear acupuncture 2006.

3. Cheng Hongfeng, Ear Acupuncture Clinical Application. 1999.

4. Zaifeng, Ear acupuncture Treatment 1999.

5. Wang Lingling, Diagram of Chinese Acupoints, 2006.